Leslie Blanchard's Hair-Coloring Book

Leslie

Hair-Coloring

by LESLIE

DOUBLEDAY & COMPANY, INC

Blanchard's Book

BLANCHARD with Zack Hanle

awings by Donald Hendricks

ARDEN CITY, NEW YORK 1982

Library of Congress Cataloging in Publication Data

Blanchard, Leslie.
    Leslie Blanchard's Hair-Coloring book.

    Includes index.
    1. Hair—Dyeing and bleaching. I. Title. II. Title:
Hair-Coloring book.
TT973.B56   646.7'242
AACR2
ISBN: 0-385-12484-8
Library of Congress Catalog Card Number 78–1181

Acknowledgments

Vermont, the state where I was born and spent my childhood, had a profound effect on my career. The naturalness of its beauty and the magnificence of the foliage colors during its changing seasons are indelibly recorded in my memory. Throughout a career that has given me just as much pleasure I have tried to duplicate this natural beauty and the subtlety of the shades nature invented.

I have also been given another gift—an understanding of what looks beautiful and glamorous—and, most of all, what makes a woman or a man feel more confident with the way she or he looks. I have been working with and studying hair, hair care and hair color for more than twenty-five years. This may seem like a long time to some, but to me it feels as if I've just begun.

I'm very proud to have had the opportunity to work with Clairol and the Gelb family, especially Bruce, with whom I have worked very closely, who have always lent me their support. My special thanks also to my friend Don Shea, and to the many editors, clients and personal friends, such as Gabriella Kalman, whose continued and total support sometimes makes me think I'm back in Vermont and this is all just a dream.

Then, a special thank-you to Barbara Walters, my friend for many years. Without her, this book would not have been written—for it was she who suggested it and encouraged me to write it to share my knowledge with others.

**Acknowledg-
ments**

Most of all, thanks to my mother and my late father, who always encouraged me to keep going even when I didn't know where I was going.

Last, my thanks to a special blonde woman who, although not in my life very long, left me with a more meaningful one.

Also, let me thank photographers Neal Barr and Jim Houghton; John Louise and John Melton, Jeffrey Rafalaf and Jack Shor of Clairol; Sara Bandy and Louis Bonadio for their makeup expertise; Richard Fowler for his hair-styling talent . . . and every one of the beautiful people who have graciously acted as role models for the Beauty Scrapbook chapter.

Leslie Blanchard

Contents

Leslie Blanchard's
Hair-Coloring Book

1

Who Needs Color?

Color is the very heart of nature; it governs our emotions, our tastes, our outlook on life.

Color is important in every phase of life—in the foods we choose to eat, in the fashions we select to wear, in decorating our homes, and in the whole of nature. Who would want to live in a black-and-gray world? Who would choose a static world, either? Change, too, is a vital keystone in the unfolding of life. Everyone needs color and change, but not always as nature dictates. You need not live with the hair color nature bestowed—and you need not have the same shade of hair for life. Just as skin and hair change with age, so do our tastes. Color is all around us, and today a myriad of hair tints and hues can almost magically be yours for the choosing.

If you were born with basically beautiful hair—vibrantly healthy, the ideal color to complement your skin and eyes, with perfect texture and manageability—you are indeed fortunate. Maintaining it as you age may be just a matter of subtly intensifying or highlighting it, while cleansing and conditioning it with care. For most people, however—both men and women —sooner or later, hair coloring becomes a desirable enhancement. Perhaps it will be only a gentle lift to give subtle brightening to fading hair. Rarely will it be an extreme, radical change of a basic color. Never should a decision to color be made impulsively, on the spur of a whimsical moment, in a fit of depression or with the idea that a drastic change will alter your whole personality or solve any major crisis in your life. What it can do is change the visual you, which in turn does wonders for the ego, the psyche and your outlook on life. Just knowing that you look better can make you feel better.

Who needs color? You do if your hair is fading to an unattractive, flat, dull lifelessness with a no-color drabness. You do if you're a natural blonde going mousy ash-blonde with no shine. Your hair may need just a bit more warmth, perhaps a hint of sunstruck gold, or merely a subtle all-over highlighting to restore light and shine and impart a honeyed glow that makes your skin and eyes come alive.

You need color if you are a true redhead whose flame has become dim and whose erstwhile radiance seems to have lost its wattage. Those darkening or fading locks can be easily restored to a beguiling red-gold shimmer with glints of new light. You need color if you're a brunette whose hair has lost its inner lights and its silken texture, and has begun to have an all-one-shade, matte appearance. It needs reviving, perhaps with a sunnier touch all over or here and there; the coloring process itself will condition its dried-out look.

You need color where there is *no color*—in the unattractive graying of some kinds of hair, in white or gray hair that has yellowish tinges, in hair that can only be described as nondescript—with no warmth, no light-and-shadow effect, and no definable hue that can be called brown or brunette, red or blonde, or variations on these, but that only can be described by such terms as "mousy," "drab," etc.

You need color if your lifestyle, your work or career, or your position in your community requires you to look your best, and yes, to look young and vital at all times. You need color if your family and friends are suggesting, "Why don't you do something with your hair?"

You need color if your hair has been over-bleached, badly colored and abused to the point where natural color has deteriorated. You need color, often only sparingly, if you are a teenager who cannot reconcile herself to what may be nature's error in the total incompatibility of her hair.

For all those reasons, hair coloring is an important—even the most important—cosmetic assistant. Beyond that, there is the often overlooked benefit of hair coloring as a corrective tool when it serves to offset facial faults. In the hands of experts, strategic placement of light and shadow in color can make a narrow face seem wider, a too-broad face appear slimmer, a low forehead look higher or a high forehead lower. Too-prominent noses or chins (and too-little chins) can be brought into more pleasing scale with careful color "shaping" and toning. Fat faces and too-round faces, flat crowns and pointy crowns, can be illusorily altered to ideal shapes with hair-coloring techniques. These feats of artistry are best left to the experts, unless the home hair-colorist is especially skillful in working with color.

You are not alone in your need for and use of hair coloring. Nearly half of the total adult female population has tried some form of rinse, tint or shampoo, in temporary or permanent form, at least once. Thanks to today's highly refined products and the skill of professional colorists, the results are ever more natural, ever more beautiful. No longer are the products harmful when properly applied, nor is the range limited, as it was several decades ago, to a basic trio of artificial colors: wild red, brass blonde and outrageous orange. There is a spectrum of choice that could permit a woman to have a change of color every day of the year. With shaping and with shading when more than one color is applied, the variations of hues are limit-less.

The almost universal acceptance of hair coloring no longer precludes a person frankly admitting that she uses it; yet for both men and women, today's techniques and products offer such natural-looking results that anyone who prefers to be secretive can easily do so. The important thing is that these nearly miraculous products be used intelligently. In the chapters that follow you will learn how best to choose and use color, and to understand why, as well as how, it works.

2

Stop! Before
You Start

Before you try a color change, analyze not only your hair, but yourself.

An architect or a great interior designer always studies not only the spaces he must fill and embellish, but also the people who will live or work there, their mode of life, their tastes, their habits and even their physical appearance. So, too, should the decision to color or recolor your hair be approached. Study yourself. Stop to analyze your own lifestyle. Ask yourself what you expect from the new color, how your present hair coloring can be improved and whether the change should be very slight or perhaps more daring.

Begin by referring to photographs taken of yourself in the last half dozen years. Even though the color will not be precise, it will give you an idea of changes in the appearance of your hair. Has it remained the same, or grown dull? Can it be improved with just a bit of highlighting, or does it need a whole new hue?

Study your hair in the mirror under bright lights. Study it outdoors in high-noon sunlight. Lift it in your fingers and look at it as the light filters through. Are you pleased with its looks and with how it feels in your hand? How it looks with your skin tone?

If you have been coloring your hair with the same formula year after year, you probably need a change, since your original hair color is constantly changing with time. As you grow older, you may have very little gray or white in your natural hair, or you may have a lot. This affects the shade of your usual hair coloring, imperceptibly at first, then increasingly more noticeably. Such a variation would strongly indicate the need for a change of your color formula.

Whether you're due for a change or you are embarking on your first adventure, take stock of your hair. Use the following chart to analyze its condition, its problems and what you have been doing to it all these years:

Hair Color

_____Natural or "virgin," never colored
_____Natural, formerly colored with permanent color
_____Natural, formerly colored with temporary color
_____Natural, formerly colored with semipermanent color
_____Colored with permanent color
_____Colored with temporary color
_____Colored with semipermanent color
_____Presently tipped, streaked or frosted
_____How often?
_____Formerly tipped, streaked or frosted
_____If semipermanent color is used, how often?
_____If permanent color is used, how often?
_____Whole head?   Retouching?
Present color of hair?_____
6   Original (natural) color?_____

Hair Health and Condition

——Normal, healthy   ——Shiny, silky   ——Good body, bouncy

Stop! Before You Start

——Oily;   ——excessively oily

——Dry;   ——dull   ——Dry, brittle, split

——Bleached, brittle, short broken ends

——Normal, healthy scalp

——Oily scalp;   ——excessively oily scalp

——Tight, tense scalp, frequently itchy

——Dry, flaky scalp   ——Dandruff

——Permanent wave

Hair Quality

——Coarse   ——Medium   ——Fine   ——Baby-fine

——Wispy   ——Average

——Thick   ——Bushy   ——Manageable

——Thin   ——Unmanageable

——Very thin   ——Balding or tending to baldness

——Very straight   ——No body   ——Good body

——Wavy   ——Slightly   ——Very

——Curly   ——Manageable   ——Unmanageable

——Too curly   ——Wiry

——Normal elasticity   ——Poor elasticity

——Over-porous   ——Nonporous   ——Normal porosity

Problems

——None

——Brow too low   ——too high

——Receding hairline   ——Irregular hairline

——Face too wide   ——too thin

——Chin too prominent   ——too small   ——receding

——Neck too long, thin   ——Neck too short   ——Fat

——Nose too prominent

——Hair grows too slowly   ——too fast

Your Overall Coloring

——Fair skin   ——Olive skin   ——Dark skin

——Very pale skin   ——Sallow skin   ——Medium-tone skin   7

——Clear skin ——Blotchy skin ——Freckles
——Oily skin ——Normal skin ——Hybrid: oily-dry
——Ruddy skin ——Pink-toned skin
Eyes: ——blue ——gray ——brown ——hazel
——other

YOUR PHYSIQUE

Height: ——Tall ——Too tall
——Medium
——Short ——Too short
Dress or suit size:——
Large-boned:—— Medium:—— Small, fine-boned:——
Weight: light—— heavy—— normal——

PRODUCTS USED ON HAIR

——Shampoo ——Cream rinse ——Conditioner
——Setting lotion ——Hair spray
——Color rinse, temporary ——Semipermanent
——Permanent color ——Color crayons
——Hair straightener
——Permanent wave: ——whole ——body ——partial

MACHINES USED ON HAIR

——Heat curlers
——Hair dryer ——salon-type ——hand-held
——blow-dryer ——comb-and-curl dryer

HAIRSTYLE

——Casual ——Classic ——Short ——Medium
——Long
——Very short ——Very long ——Wavy ——Curly
——Frizzy ——Chignon ——Formal ——Variable
——Current and mainstream ——Current and faddy

LIFESTYLE

——Active, outdoor person ——Indoor

——General health is: ——good ——fair ——poor

——Allergies (specify):————————————————
——Wear hats: ——often ——sometimes ——never
——Wear scarves: ——often ——sometimes ——never   *Stop! Before*
——Wish to look older ——younger ——your age   *You Start*
——Wear tailored fashions
——Prefer soft, feminine fashions
——Like both, as the occasion demands

The Calendar

Your birthday (year):————————
Last hairstyling change:———————— coloring change:——————
Last hair trim, shaping or cut:————————
Last conditioning treatment:————————
Last permanent:———————— or hair straightening:————————
Last shampoo:————————
Today's date:————————

With this complete profile of you and your hair, you're ready to find the hair color you should have. Your hair basically fits in one of the categories of color in this book—blonde, brownette, brunette, red or gray. Turn to your chapter first for how to lighten, brighten, shade or darken. If you are considering a complete color change, read through all the different categories before making your decision. Bear in mind, however, that you are constantly changing with the years. Flaxen blonde in your teens doesn't mean flaxen blonde at thirty-plus. Very dark shades are unbecoming to older faces, which need the enhancement and brightening of light. White hair, properly cared for, can be dazzling, and prematurely gray hair is often flattering, but dull gray hair flatters no one, young or old.

Your hair, before being colored, must be in optimum condition. If necessary, take time for some thorough conditioning treatments—deep ones that stay in the hair for at least twenty minutes. Massage with your fingertips (the balls of the fingers) to make sure that the scalp is relaxed and that there are no   *9* dry, flaky patches on it. Use a cream conditioner and wrap your hair in hot towels (soaked in hot water and wrung out) two or three times. Then rinse in cool water (never hot) and either let the hair dry naturally (the ideal way) or with a cool dryer. All this should take place two or three days before you undertake coloring.

Hair should not be colored when it's extremely soiled, but neither should it be colored when it's been freshly shampooed —especially if your scalp tends to be sensitive. If a shampoo is necessary for cleanliness, do it a day or two before coloring, and use just a light, gentle cleanser that won't strip the hair of its natural oil film. A good shampoo usually has a creamy base that cleans the hair and the scalp without leaving its own coating on the hair and without leaving the hair so stripped that it becomes fly-away and full of static when it is dry. Never use bar soap, and don't feel that lots of suds mean a super shampoo. Some of the best simply form a creamy lather. Choose your shampoo by reading labels carefully; buy the one that is for your hair type—oily, dry, normal or color-treated. Always rinse conditioners and shampoos out of the hair with cool water. Rinse with a downward motion, using your fingers as a wide-toothed comb. Never rub and scrub dry. Just squeeze excess moisture out through the towel and pat rather than rub the strands. Run your fingers through the hair and gently shake the strands, then pat until dripping ceases. Let your hair dry naturally in the air whenever possible. Always handle your hair as if it were a fine fabric—silk or cashmere or any other fine fiber.

Before you start to color, check your chart. Has your hair had any chemical treatments of any kind, such as a permanent wave or straightening? If this has been done recently, wait until after one or two shampoos and a conditioning treatment before coloring your hair. These chemical processes make the hair much more absorbent; therefore, if coloring must take

place, the coloring agent itself must be diluted with water and left on for less time than usual. Otherwise the color will "grab" the hair shafts too quickly, and will look heavy and deeper-toned on the ends.

Whether you're a long-time user of hair color—in the salon or at home—or a tentative first-timer, take time to select the right color for you. If it looks obvious, it's wrong—and mistakes are hard to correct. Used properly so that the results are natural looking, hair coloring is one of the greatest of all beauty aids for creating an attractive aura.

3

Your Coloring Scrapbook

It is shading and the reflection of light, the many blendings of different colors, that make hair coloring so different and so natural today.

What you see in the mirror under the bathroom light is *not* the way others see you. So, for a more realistic look at yourself, your hair and your makeup, have a series of color snapshots taken. Comb your hair differently for each photograph, try different kinds of makeup and show full-face, three-quarter face and profile. Change blouses or tops to find out which colors and lines are most flattering to your face and hair. Have some full-length pictures snapped; your overall look is important, too, in selecting a hairstyle and color. These will all be your "before" pictures for your hair and beauty scrapbook. After studying the pictures, you are ready to move forward.

Take them to your hair stylist and your colorist when you decide to change your look. Or, if conditioning and coloring are such that you can do these jobs yourself, study the pictures carefully to see whether your hair should go lighter or darker, be merely highlighted after intensive conditioning, or just receive an overall highlighting and conditioning rinse.

In the color photographs, you will see the case histories of eight women, from the teen years to maturity, and how these women changed their looks from rather ordinary to lively, exciting and sparkling beauty. These are, as we say, "real people," like you and me. In each case, you will see three pictures of each—a "before," a shampooed-and-conditioned semistyled hairdo, and a final, color-treated and fully styled coif. The makeup in each photograph remains the same, so that the full impact of hair coloring and healthier hair is emphasized as the key to looking infinitely more attractive. The effects of good conditioning are readily visible in each case, with hair looking more fluid and bouncier, reflecting light and color, and coming alive because it is healthier.

Study these "case histories." Decide which direction and course of action you wish to take. Remember: what looked pretty at fifteen doesn't at forty. Different ages demand not only different kinds of coloring, but different hairstyles and different care.

If you need help, take your own collection of photographs and this book to your stylist and your colorist; then confer and decide together, which is the best change and the most beautiful for you.

4

Color You Blonde

Blonde hair must be pampered to be beautiful and believable. It is not just one color, but a thousand delicate, shining shades, from light to dark.

Blonde is probably the color I'm most well known for, but do you think I have a favorite color? I'm not telling, or at least not yet—but blonde is certainly a color that fits and complements the widest range of people.

The fairy-tale princess is always a blonde; the Lorelei, mermaids, Eve, and Botticelli's Venus were all blondes; gentlemen prefer them. They have been symbols of purity in legend and lore; sex symbols since the flapper era of the Twenties. They have been labeled "classic," "cool," "patrician" and "sunny." In any case, it seems to be true that not only do "blondes have more fun," they *are* more fun. Ask the woman who is one—or, better yet, the woman who has just become one.

What *is* this blonde mystique? It is centuries old, but in this country it may have started in motion pictures, when Mary
Pickford, with her golden curls, became "America's Sweet-

heart." Since most Caucasian children are born blonde, mothers by the millions began trying to keep their daughters blonde with a variety of home concoctions, from herbs and teas to lemon juice. The success of Shirley Temple gave further impetus to the blonde-and-curly craze. There followed a succession of stars, from sophisticated to sexy, who kept the blonde ball rolling: Dolores Costello, Lilyan Tashman, Greta Garbo, Jean Harlow, Ann Harding, Joan Blondell, Sonja Henie, Veronica Lake, Carole Lombard, Mae West, Betty Grable, Lana Turner, Marlene Dietrich, Ingrid Bergman, Carroll Baker, Grace Kelly and, finally, the irreplaceable Marilyn Monroe, who once said, "I like to feel blonde all over."

Very few early stars were natural blondes; many featured nearly white or platinum shades, achieved with the hair-destroying harsh bleaches of the time. The rage for blonde stars in the early days of film-making was logical from a movie producer's viewpoint: blondes were more photogenic than brunettes because their hair reflected light, while dark hair simply soaked it up and would look flat. Today, however, despite more advanced lighting and camera techniques, blonde models and actresses are still the most popular. In fact, they are more so than ever, since the best blondes have hair shaded and toned with such subtlety and artistry that it offers an infinity of light and color play under the camera and to the eye.

Helping to popularize the blonde look by virtue of stunningly attractive hair today are such stars and models as Catherine Deneuve, Dina Merrill, Candice Bergen, Cheryl Tiegs, Farrah Fawcett, Meryl Streep, Lauren Hutton, Cheryl Ladd and Nancy Allen. Among these, no two are alike, which is the way of the world of blondes today, so wide is the color range, so varied are the placements of highlights and tones. Thanks to the wealth of excellent products for creating and maintaining light hair, a blonde can be as unique as her fingerprints and much more changeable. One sees less and less breakage and hair damage on blonde heads compared to the platinum-and-bleach era of Jean Harlow and Mae West. Only bad judgment and carelessness result in such offenses as dark-at-the-roots blonde hair, brassy blondeness, straw-textured and frizzy blondeness, or drab, dull blondeness.

Perhaps our attraction to blonde hair is that when it is beautiful, truly beautiful, it appears to have snared a bit of the sun, and sunlight makes everyone happy. In every hue and combination of shades, and for almost every age, blonde hair brightens the face and brings out one's best features. Its soft play of light is the ultimate in flattery for the complexion. The mature beauties of the world know this—Princess Grace, Lauren Bacall, Alexis Smith, Joan Fontaine, Dina Merrill, and that dazzling model of the Forties, Sunny Harnett. As their years increase, their blondeness keeps them youthful and soft as no other hair color can.

How many ways can you be blonde? As noted, the shades are legion. Just look at the numbers and the names of blonde hair colorings on the shelf of your store. There are such chic names as pear, champagne, honey and innocent. This is what makes them totally believable: hair color is makeup for the hair, and blonde coloring must be done with the greatest of taste and simplicity.

There are descriptive names: ash, sunlit beige, honey, strawberry blonde, moonglow, sandy and the like. There are poetic and romantic and whimsical names. Each company has its own, and the search for new names is as wide as it is for makeup colors. Often the name is no clue to the color, and one must study color charts carefully, although a printed color is only a close approximation of how it will appear on the hair. Printed colors are opaque and flat; hair has translucence and vitality. With the newer, more-natural-than-ever way of coloring the hair, you may have not one, but several colors of blonde all at once. After all, natural blondes have many different colors throughout their hair. No longer is it possible to categorize blondes with specific color names. You are or will be, depending on your eyes and complexion, a warm, medium-warm, dark warm (which I think looks best with brown or hazel eyes), medium or cool blonde (which highlights blue or gray-green eyes). In addition, you can be called a light, medium or dark blonde. After that, the individual nuances of shading and highlighting will give you your own unique, one-of-a-kind blondeness.

Creating the most delicate, the palest blondes, which call for prelightening and then the application of extra-delicate tints and toners, is an intricate business which really calls for a colorist's advice. So, too, is the complex artistry of duplicating nature through the dimension-illusion of light and shadow from brow to nape (where hair is naturally darker because of heavier deposits of oil glands). Some hair coloring is easier to do at home, but a radical change is not advisable—from very dark to light, for example. For the woman who is dark blonde wishing to go lighter, or a light blonde whose hair is fading or graying and who wishes to be a warmer, livelier blonde, there are dozens of conditioner-fortified products that do the job— either temporarily (from shampoo to shampoo), semiper-manently or permanently. There are also highlighting tricks she can do herself (see Special Effects, Chapter 9) or have done at the salon, depending on the style and on the time available. These include sun streaks, achieved by selecting strands around the face to lighten; "painting" (see Glossary) strands for nature-duplicating color, or adding a haze of highlights by selecting strands for lightening over most of the head.

Whatever you choose to do in the blonde realm, go gently, go cautiously and go gradually if you are uncertain. Less is best on the first try. Reach your goal in slow, easy stages. Try a temporary color rinse first; you can always wash it out. It will not penetrate the hair shafts but will lie on the outer surface of the hair. With fairly light hair you can achieve a golden blonde, but with darker blondes, only golden highlights will be added. To brighten natural blondes and blend in early

17

gray hair, the semipermanent colors work nicely, fading gradually after several shampoos.

Permanent, one-step-process blonde shades will lighten the hair, color the gray or white hairs, and add body and better texture to the hair. They will make dark blondes lighter and you can add many subtle shades as well so your hair looks more natural. For brown or dark brown mixed with gray, double-process or two-step blonding is necessary. This involves prelightening, then toning. Carefully selected strands toned different shades, starting lighter in the front and gradually darkening as you go backward, will make your hair the most beautiful and naturally exciting blonde possible. In effect, this is custom coloring, and it requires an expert's skill.

In any case, if you go blonde at home, and this is a first attempt, be sure to do a Patch Test (see Glossary) first, and also a Strand Test (see Glossary) to determine the shade you want. Snip off several strands from unobtrusive parts of the head—from near the face, on the crown, at the nape. Color these according to the manufacturer's directions; let them dry. If still unsure, seek additional advice before you start. Look at the strands of hair on a sheet of white paper, first in strong sunlight, then under normal indoor lighting. Hold them against your skin. If the color isn't right for you, stop right there and choose another. If you think it is what you want, or nearly so, cover your hair with a scarf, make up your lips and eyes to go with the new color and again hold the test strands against your face—near the brow and at the sides—under strong light. Will it work? If so, go ahead. Go blonde in the shade of your choice.

Once you have become a blonde, by choice or even by birth, you have a commitment and must live up to being blonde. Almost more than any other color, except gray or white, it requires special care. Just the atmosphere, the everyday dirt from the air, can play havoc with it, but you can't shampoo too often. Always use gentle or delicate shampoos designed especially for blondes whose hair has been lightened, tinted or shaded. You will need special added conditioners to keep your hair from getting dry and brittle and to keep the color from fading. If you cover your hair while in sunlight, be sure that straw hats and cotton scarves are loose; repeated snug coverings can produce excessive perspiration, which could cause color damage. Keep your hair loosely styled; its greatest beauty is light filtering through it as it moves. Dark roots must never be allowed to appear; if you haven't the time to prevent this, then you will be better off with a dark blonde, or even a golden-brown color with highlights. Faithful hair-shaping and styling is a must, even if it is only a matter of trimming ends as they grow to keep them smooth, silky and controlled.

You, the newly blonde, must be blonde through and through. You are now the fairy-tale princess or the glamorous lovely of your dreams: your clothes, your accessories, your makeup must be keyed to your style and type of blondeness. Soon this selectivity will be part of you, second nature, and you won't have to be constantly in a puzzle about what designs, fabrics and colors are best for you. You can live up to your hair effortlessly, as if you had the greatest hairdresser possible.

BLONDE Q'S AND A'S

Just what does prelightening do to the hair? Isn't it really bleaching, and can't it do harm to the hair?

Bleaching is an old-fashioned word which was used in the days when the agents were ammonia and peroxide, with no conditioning elements. Even more old-fashioned was the word "blanching." Prelightening is not as strong as bleaching; all of the pigment is not taken out of the hair. There is no hint of ammonia and the peroxide used in the formulas should never be stronger than 20 percent V.N.V. If your scalp is at all sen-

sitive, use a cream developer (see Glossary). It is but one of
the helpful ingredients of today's gentle lightening products.
For brown and dark brown hair to successfully receive the
shade or tone desired, it must first be lightened to a specific
degree; i.e., the natural pigment of the hair is removed. The
stages of decoloration can range from deep yellow for a very
dark blonde, to yellow for a medium blonde, to light yellow
for a light blonde. The lightener is left on longest for dark
hair going to the palest blonde. The prelightening procedure
also serves to make the hair shaft more porous, so that the subsequent toner will readily penetrate and remain in the hair.
Strong, resistant hair will take longer to prelighten. Even if
your hair is dark and mixed with white, it should be prelightened for the necessary porosity. After the prelightener is shampooed out, your hair is immediately treated to a hair- and
scalp-nourishing conditioner. This, too, is rinsed out and a *filler*
is applied before any actual color is introduced into the hair
(see Glossary). The depth of the filler depends on the
lightness or depth of the blonde color desired. Each step is a
protective one, ensuring the health of the hair and actually
reinforcing weak, damaged or fine hair so that it will hold on
to the color longer. Properly executed, the process in no way
hurts the hair; on the contrary, it restores it to new vitality,
giving it more body and manageability along with the color
enhancement. The cleansing and conditioning steps leave the
scalp glowing; those who have their hair properly prelightened
and toned almost never play hostess to dandruff and itchy
scalp.

*What is the cap method for frosting and streaking hair, and
is it a good idea?*

The hair is combed down all around and a snug-fitting plastic
cap dotted all over with small holes is placed over it and tied
securely under the chin. With a crochet hook, small strands
are pulled through the holes all over the head or in selected

areas for strategic placing of streaks. These strands are then lightened while the remaining hair is left untouched. This process is done to control the extent of the lightening effect you want. Another and sometimes better way is to pick out strands and wrap them in aluminum foil after they are treated to a lightening agent, which is left on for whatever time is necessary to produce the desired effect. When the foil is removed, the hair is shampooed, toned to produce a more natural highlighted look and then conditioned. Both of these methods can produce streaks, a light haze around the hairline and face or an all-over night-lighted effect.

Is hair spray all right to use on blonde hair, especially the kind that has flyaway, unmanageable wisps?

Yes, but only the very gentle, finest spray should be used. Gems don't sparkle when they aren't clean; similarly, blonde hair needs the utmost care to keep shining. Just a drop of light moisturizing cream worked with the palms of your hands and then stroked on the hair lightly does the trick of controlling flyaway hair.

Sometimes blonde hair begins to turn unpleasantly orange or brassy several weeks after it has been colored. What causes this, and what can be done to eliminate it?

This was a common complaint years ago, but is much less so with the present-day color formulas, color-protecting shampoos and conditioners. There are special rinses for toning down the offensive brassy color. These are temporary and are applied after shampooing, conditioning, rinsing and towel-drying the hair. Look for rinses described as "cool white" or "ash"—but do not make a steady practice of using these, because they do have a slightly dulling and drabbing effect.

How often should blonde hair be retouched?

Depending on the rate of growth of the individual's hair, the degree of lightness of the blonde hair and the degree of darkness of the original hair, this can vary from about once a month to six weeks, but never longer. The new natural shadings, using several tones of blonde, make regrowth far less obvious than the old-fashioned, all-one-color blonde. Letting it go too long, however, doesn't help the hair. Remember, a beautiful blonde is always a fresh blonde.

Is there anything on the market that will camouflage growing-out dark roots on lightened hair?

There are a few fool-the-eye tricks that can carry you over until your hair can be redone, but remember: What you see, everyone else sees, too. Wear a softer, looser hairdo. Smooth, close-to-the-head styles make the roots more obvious, especially if the hair is fine or thin. Wear a partless style and fluff the hair around the hairline to make regrowth less visible. A dry shampoo sprayed near the roots and then blended in can camouflage dark roots the best.

How can hair be kept looking attractive while the blonding grows out and the hair returns to its natural shade?

The hair may be tinted to match or blend with its original shade, leaving some highlights of blonde. An alternative is to use a temporary rinse that blends with the natural hair, until the hair can be trimmed. If for any reason you want a complete rest from all coloring, for health reasons or for the hair's condition, then the practical and logical solution is to cover it with a good wig.

What causes lightened hair to look greenish?

Too much ash in the toner. Chemicals in swimming pools, and even salt water, also can have this effect if the hair isn't thoroughly rinsed in clear water after a swim. Sometimes, too, coloring hair that has a henna rinse or a metallic rinse on it can
cause a greenish tint to appear.

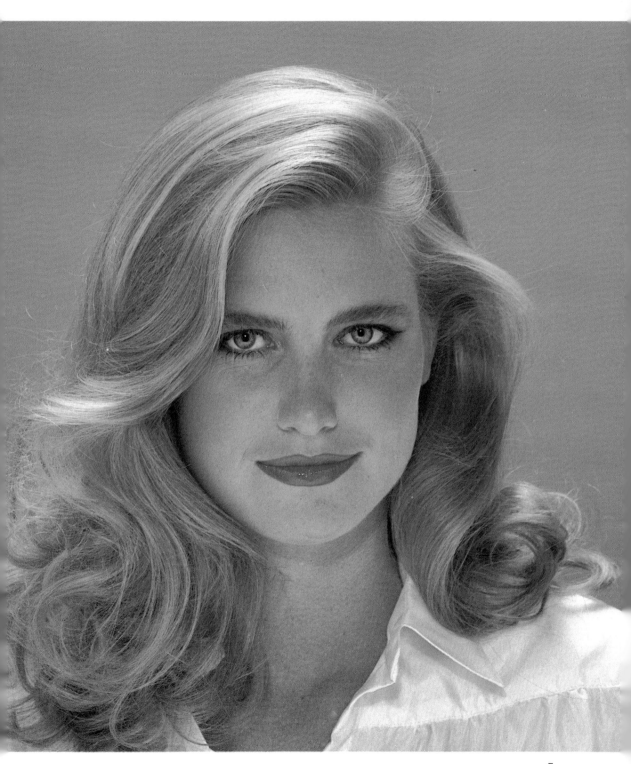

The ultimate blonde. (Photo by Harold Kreiger, courtesy Clairol)

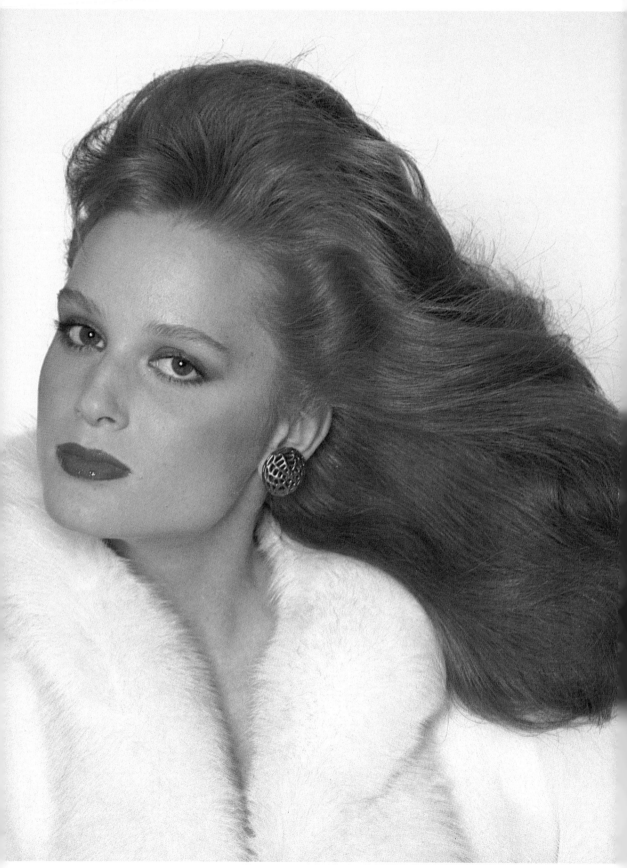

2   The ultimate redhead. (Photo by Neal Barr, courtesy Clairol)

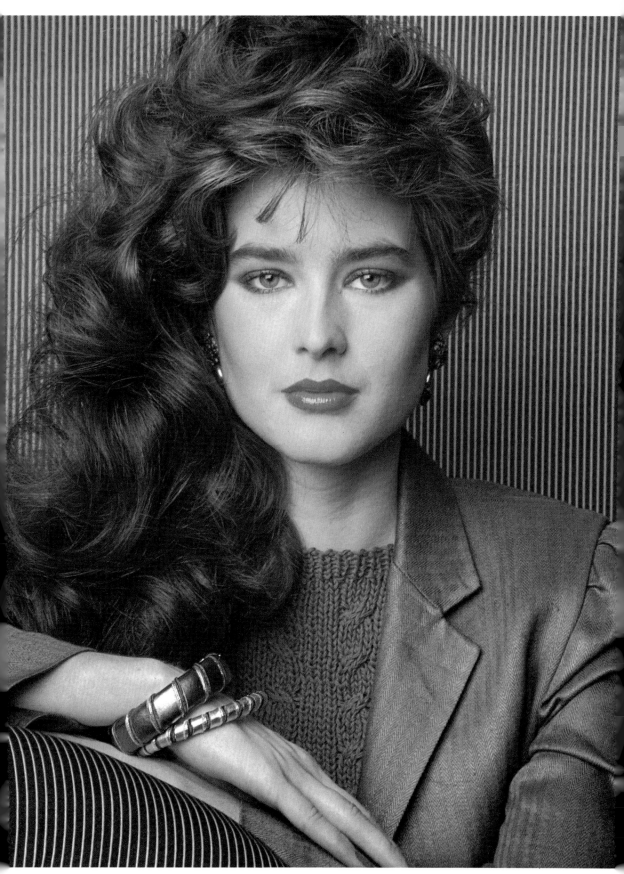

The ultimate brownette. (Photo by Neal Barr, courtesy Clairol) 3

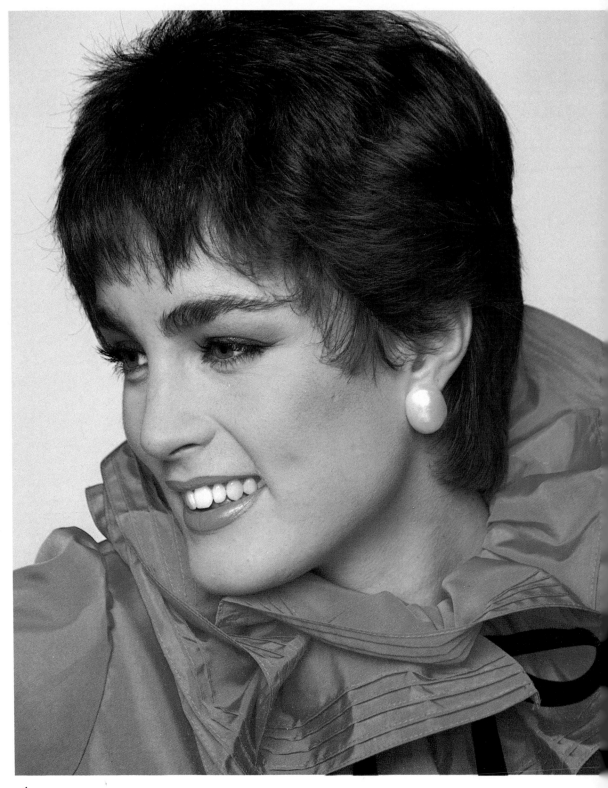

4   The ultimate brunette. (Photo by Neal Barr, courtesy Clairol)

Should the hair be shampooed before coloring?

This is not necessary; often it is better not to shampoo. All coloring agents have a cleansing property; besides, vestiges of your own preshampooing on your hair might interfere with the coloring process or affect certain sensitive scalps.

How can one determine if the hair has been over-lightened?

The best way is when it's wet. It will be almost impossible to comb, have little elasticity, mat easily and feel almost gummy to the touch.

How can over-lightened hair be corrected?

If it is in very bad shape, give it a rest from lighteners, toners and permanents or relaxers. Use rinses only until hair is in better condition. Have a series of deep conditioning treatments and have as many of the damaged ends as possible trimmed. When hair is extremely damaged it has no moisture and will break easily.

Is it normal for lighteners to burn or sting the scalp?

Not unless you have a very sensitive scalp, have been ill or are extremely tense. Any nicks, cuts or abrasions on the scalp should be coated with petroleum jelly, since these could cause a stinging sensation. If the hair has been lightened repeatedly with the same product and a sudden burning reaction occurs, a sensitivity may have developed from medication or a chemical imbalance in your body. Some women cannot use lighteners within a day or two preceding their menstrual cycle. A patch test on very pale or delicate skins should be made to see if there is a sensitivity; if so, lightening should be discontinued for a while until a subsequent patch test shows no reaction.

Is it possible to become allergic to a lightener or a tint?

This rarely occurs. An allergic reaction means that something has triggered your sensitivity button and tipped the allergy balance of your body. This rarely happens with tints or toners and lighteners today. One may develop a sensitivity, as noted, although with today's gentle, creamy lighteners, so fortified with conditioning agents, this rarely happens. If it does occur, contact your physician and have a checkup; thyroid conditions, diabetes and certain medications can cause temporary sensitivity.

What are the so-called "seven stages" of hair lightening?

Each manufacturer has instructions in the bleaching products to describe what this means. If there is something you don't understand after reading them, a toll-free number is often given on the package to clarify additional questions.

How are silver and platinum shades obtained?

Only after extreme prelightening to the palest yellow of the seven stages can a silver toner be applied. Unfortunately, many are very unbecoming and dated-looking. I don't recommend them. They do not look natural.

How long before hair is lightened can it be permanent-waved or straightened?

Ideally, no less than two weeks before. At the very least, a week before.

Are lighteners applied to wet hair?

No. Best results are obtained when they are applied to dry hair.

How long should lighteners be left on the hair?

Again, manufacturers have guidelines in their bleaching and toning products. Follow these very closely. Color, the natural porosity of the hair and the coarseness or fineness of the hair are all factors dictating the amount of time necessary to lighten hair to the proper stage for receiving a tint or toner. All this varies with the individual, which is why the hair should be checked frequently to find the ideal moment when the lightener should be removed and its action discontinued. Keep an accurate record and you should find that the results are consistent.

Can eyebrows be lightened and toned to match or complement the hair with the same lightener and toner that has been used on the hair?

This is possible, but is not advisable as a job for the amateur. All coloring agents and lighteners bear warning labels that caution against getting products in or near the eyes. Even with the eye area coated with a protective cream or jelly, it is difficult to lighten brows with the eyes closed. It is far better to have a beautician do this for you, in states where it is permitted by law. The brows should not be as light as the paler blondes, but a few shades darker.

At what age should one stop being a blonde?

Never—but, naturally, a different blonde color may be more flattering. Once there were very few blondes over forty. Today, the older woman can actually benefit from the lighter colors framing her face. Today's softer, gentler shadings of blonde are more natural-looking on older women as long as they are not too pale.

Is it all right to use lighteners on a blonde-going-brunette child's hair?

Using adult products to lighten a child's hair is never advisable. Young people's hair is usually much more fragile and young scalps much more tender than grown-ups'. There will be products on the market suited for young people.

Does lightening the hair cause dandruff?

Never. Dandruff is a scalp disease. If it exists before the hair is lightened, it may be checked, but not cured, by the cleansing action of the lightener. The white flakes that appear after repeated lightening signal excessive dryness of the scalp.

What causes some parts of the hair to lighten more than others?

Natural hair is never all one color. Surface hair, exposed to the sun and artificial light, is lighter than the hair underneath. Hair around the temples and the sides of the brow is frequently lighter than the rest, and hair at the nape is usually darkest of all. If a lightening agent is evenly distributed over the entire head for the same length of time, there will be the same lighter and darker areas that nature bestowed. This can be attractive in the final toning because it will be more natural than having all one color with no lights and shadows. If the lights and darks of nature are too contrasty, lightener should be applied to the unacceptably dark areas first. This allows a few more minutes of lightening before the remaining hair is treated, thereby making the two shades more compatible.

FASHION AND BEAUTY CUES

If your hair has been more than just a little lightened—if you've gone from brown to blonde—then you must make a whole new appraisal of the colors you're wearing on your lips, your skin and your eyes. Your wardrobe needs close scrutiny, too, in the light of your new blondeness. Start first with makeup; you'll want to wear the new shades when you go forth to select complementary clothing replacements if necessary.

The basic rule for all kinds and types of blonde makeup is: go easy, go lightly. Blondes require the subtlest makeup—no bold slashes of too-bright lipstick, no heavy eye liners and brow colorings, no eye shadows in very strong shades, and never, never such intense blushers that the effect is that of a painted doll. For today's wonderfully natural-looking blondes, makeup that looks softly natural and blended is the most complementary. Makeup colors can be a bit more intense for evening, but never so overpowering as to detract from the main feature of the show—your shiningly wonderful blonde hair. Its color and its light play make it your most important accessory. Learn to use it like an accessory, especially at night. Make it festive by lifting it softly and looping it or twining it to frame the face or gathering it low on the nape of your neck in a shining chignon. Handle it like fine fabric—a silk scarf that can be worn many ways to create the mood you want.

Of course, blondes have many choices, but there are special looks I prefer for each type. The pale, cool blonde with a patrician look, whose hair is highlighted with a soft rose-gold color, is flattered by simplicity of line in fashion. Hers are the no-frills clothes in pure, uncluttered colors—turquoise, apple green, sea blue, white (and black is always exciting) for evenings. She may wear her hair more sleekly than most, with a wide, sweeping curve or a single furl of soft, open curl around the ends. Her skin is creamy, with a gentle flush of light rose blusher worn high on the cheeks. Eyelashes and eye liner are medium brown, with a soft charcoal mascara. Lips may be touched with a deep rose or a glowing raspberry or other tones in that realm—with a soft sheen, but never too shiny.

The Scandinavian, outdoorsy blonde, with golden wheat-color hair and an almost perpetual rosy-tan complexion, wears her hair in a swinging long bob and needs little blusher. She should never date her looks with makeup. Lips may be glossed with a light rose-pink in a clear, natural way. Her close sister, the California blonde, has the same healthy outdoor look, but her blondeness is warmer, sunnier, and her locks are worn in a tumble of waves and loose, open curls that catch and reflect the light with every movement of her head. She is the sun-kissed blonde, with warm-toned skin flushed with a peach-to-amber blush and the same ripe peach tone more intensely on her lips. Her eye liner is there, but gently, in a golden brown that intensifies for her mascara. She opts for casual fashions and the sportswoman look.

The fragile or come-take-care-of-me blonde chooses romantic hairdos, especially for evening, with clutches of curls tied or pinned with pretty hair accessories. Her skin is delicate, ivory to almost-white, and she flushes it ever-so-lightly with a matte, rose-petal-soft pink blusher that looks like the inside of a seashell. Her mouth wears clear, light pink lipstick, never too shiny, and her brows are feathered with the lightest of browns. If her eyes are blue or gray, she may use a light blue shadow for emphasis. Hers are the romantic clothes—the sheer, fragile, feminine blouses and fluid, airy fabrics.

Blonde hair can be worn with every eye color, from blue to gray to brown in all its shades. As I mentioned before, brown is one of the most exciting eye colors with blonde hair, if the accompanying skin tones are not sallow.

So varied are the shades of blonde today that one no longer labels them. The range goes from the coolest and palest to the dark-blonde borderline brownette and the strawberry-blonde borderline redhead. Highlighting and shading are today's keys to achieving these new, exciting tones. The blonde's only problem in fashion is that when certain shock colors, muddy tones or wildly exotic purples and lacquer reds make news as the latest fad, she must detour and choose more complementary colors for her golden look. The same is true for makeup fashions that look harsh, unnatural and faddish.

BLONDE DO'S AND DON'TS

Do show blonde at its best. Keep blonde hairstyling light, airy, soft, so that its play of highlights can be shown to advantage.

DON'T wear plastered-down, tightly pinned-back hairdos. Avoid skin-tight pony tails, braids and pigtails. These will make hair look darker and show roots. Blonde hair is the most fragile in many cases, and these hairstyles can cause breakage if worn constantly.

Don't permanent-wave over newly blonded hair. Wait several weeks, or a week or two before recoloring. Waving and straightening chemicals can alter the delicate toning and even cause unwanted brassiness.

Don't overbrush hair. Grandmother's one hundred strokes are no longer the rule. Too much and too vigorous brushing can harm the hair shafts. Never brush hair when it's wet; hair is at its lowest tensile strength and most vulnerable to breakage when it is wet. Use a conditioner that needs no rinsing out, to strengthen and protect your hair.

Do be meticulous about conditioning and cleansing blonde hair. Surface dirt, air pollutants and dust from the atmosphere make light hair look especially dull and dirty.

Don't use lighteners and toners if the scalp is sore, abraded, or showing any symptoms of disease. Wait until cuts and bruises have healed and the scalp is in healthy condition.

Don't let lighteners and toners overlap when you color again. Not only will there be demarcation lines at the regrowth area—often a solid band or ring—but breakage can occur.

Do use conditioners on the hair after it has been lightened. It will make the texture of the hair uniform, and color will shine and look very fresh. Conditioners still should be used after every cleansing, since they remove unwanted oil, add manageability and shine, and remove any trace of shampoo that would dull hair if left in.

Do choose and use blonde-hair care products carefully. Shampoos for lightened and delicate hair, conditioners for the same and hair sprays, if they are used lightly, keep blonde hair brilliant. Follow the directions to the letter for these and all hair products—especially coloring formulas.

Don't use home-brewed products for conditioning; harsh bleaches, ammonia or peroxide mixtures of your own should not be applied in an attempt to lighten hair. Hair-care companies spend a lot of money and time perfecting conditioners for you, so you don't have to be a chemist. Do dry hair naturally whenever you have the time, in the fresh air, and never scrub it dry with a towel. Minimize use of hot curlers as a constant curling aid, and never use blowers and dryers at the highest setting.

Do cleanse hair in tepid water. Never rinse or condition or shampoo in hot water.

Don't set hair on metal rollers or with bobby pins, especially if the hair is a very light, fine, delicate blonde. Every roller and pin mark will leave a line. Use smooth plastic rollers with plastic pics and don't stretch the hair too tightly when setting it. Never sleep on settings; this only increases the chances of having fishhook curls with bent ends. Never go to bed with wet hair. This is not conducive to good health and, in the case of delicate blonde hair, will cause it to dry in all kinds of unmanageable shapes.

Don't apply lightener to the entire head of hair during retouching. Protect the previously lightened hair with a bit of creamy conditioner to avoid overlap.

Do wear blonde hair shorter as time goes by, even though it is most often associated with long bobs. Softly waved and fluffed blonde hair is more becoming to the woman in her later years. Even a short-short cut with open curls can be more flattering on the older woman than the downward lines of long hair.

Don't use a cap or a hair dryer to speed up or activate lightening processes.

Do choose blonde coloring with an eye to your skin tones. Go just a step or two lighter at first if you're aiming at extremely light hair, and remember that it's most beautiful on the young. Women with yellowish or olive complexions look best in the darker tones of blonde. Creamy- or ivory-skinned women can almost range the whole gamut of blonde. Ruddy or deep pink skins should avoid colors with red or red-gold in them. After a certain age, lighter is best, since light hair makes the complexion look fresher, brighter and younger. However, too-light hair can make you older looking if it gets a white or gray cast.

DON'T leave lighteners on the hair any longer than necessary; make frequent strand tests to check the stage of coloring.

DON'T use metal bowls or tools when tinting or lightening. Use plastic bowls, measurers, applicators and other utensils. Always wear protective gloves.

Do work under proper lighting. Clear north daylight is best for selecting and applying color. Use incandescent rather than fluorescent light; the latter is inclined to give a bluish and grayish cast and masks reds and golds.

5

Color You Red

From the palest strawberry blonde to deep, glowing auburn, red is the liveliest of all hair colors and requires more meticulous care than any other.

Psychologically, red is never an in-between color; people either love it or hate it. Born redheads have often been buffeted by unwelcome nicknames in their childhood—"carrot top," "brick top" or just plain "red." Later they are called "spitfire," "crazy redhead" and, sometimes, "witchy." However, as with brunettes, who are frequently said to be sullen or sultry, and blondes, who are sometimes labeled "dumb," it is pure myth that flaming hair signifies an inflammable disposition. Hair color is never a clue to an individual's temperament.

Richest and rarest of all hair hues, red in its many shades has been prized through the ages. Immortalized by the painter Titian, red-gold tresses were so coveted by aristocratic Venetian ladies that they suffered tedious hours and endless, often harmful concoctions in efforts to achieve the elusive "titian" locks.

Hair was sponged with solutions of black sulfur, soda and

alum, then dried in the sun. Henna packs of a special harshness were popular and least damaging, though comparatively ineffectual, as were various tea rinses. All this was done for the love of red hair, which seems, in the language of fashion, to be always "in." From ancient times to the present, both Greece and Italy have favored red hair. During the reign of Good Queen Bess (who was a sandy redhead) Elizabethans admired red—provided by nature or artifice—as the fashionable hair color. In America, with the advent of color movies, the most sought-after actresses were those with reddish-gold or strawberry-blonde hair. Then and now, some of our most celebrated beauties are famous for their flaming tresses—Maureen O'Hara, Arlene Dahl, Rita Hayworth, Suzy Parker, Patty Hanson, Lucille Ball, Gertrude Lawrence, Maggie Smith, Ann-Margret, Jane Fonda and scores more.

The spectrum of reds is extremely broad, since red is not a single shade, but many. In nature it ranges from nearly blonde to nearly brown, as in the dark auburn Sophia Loren. Simple highlighting of the warm-toned, reddish browns adds further shades. Still more can be added with the tints and tones manufactured today, to extend the range almost to infinity.

If you decide to improve on nature or to enhance your natural color with something from the red spectrum, you must first determine what kind of redhead you are—or hope to be. Study your skin tones, the color of your eyes, the shade of your hair. Are you or do you plan to be a *strawberry blonde?* This is the lightest shade of all, full of golden lights and very nearly blonde. The skin coloring that accompanies this shade is like that of a dark blonde. It is usually unfreckled, fair and creamy. The pale, almost white skin is ethereally beautiful with this shade. Eyes are usually light—gray, green or blue. The light, *bright redhead* most often has a pale complexion, leaning toward a pinkish tone that blushes easily. Eyes are usually blue, sometimes green. Freckles appear most often with this combination. The *coppery redhead*—a light auburn—

sports vivid, intensely colored tresses with a skin that varies from pale and freckled through creamy pale to the so-called medium complexion. Eyes are blue, hazel, green or gray. The *deepest auburn*, including a nearly *brown mahogany* type, varies in skin type as the coppery redhead does. Now and then the darker redheads have brown eyes, which are extremely rare with the lighter shades of red.

The tones of redheads should all be within the golden, amber or coppery shades, to look natural and to be becoming. When they begin to look pink or purple they seem very artificial, very unnatural, adding an almost yellow, unflattering cast to the skin. True copper tones add softness and give the skin a healthier, pinkish glow. By copper we mean the shine of a bright new penny—with golden highlights.

Born reds, as time goes by, need assistance to keep tresses light, airy and touched with gold. Age darkens the highlights, fades the palest reds and dulls the sheen. The few who are born with brilliant orangey-red hair find that it gradually darkens as they grow older. Natural red hair will have strands of all the colors, from blonde and brown to almost a gray-brown, mixed with the red. The lightest, almost blonde reds tend to have hair that is very fine, silky and delicate. This type of hair needs special care with the gentlest of shampoos and conditioners to maintain its attractiveness. The Irish-setter type of red, an almost chestnut red with touches of brown, is thicker and coarser. This type grows darker with age, becoming more brownette. To keep it lovely, it should be lightened. The lightening should be very subtle, on the golden side, never resulting in the purple-maroon-burgundy colors, which are very dramatic and belong to very young, trendy people. The color to strive for as auburn hair ages is more red, but with golden brown in it, always keeping it soft with highlights, especially around the face. As time goes by, the skin becomes softer, paler, and red hair also should become softer.

In choosing formulas to color you red, it is always best to

use a golden color in combination with the deep, reddish shades. This will keep it light, soft and airy. Usually you need the next color lighter than what you've been using, because dark reds go almost brown as they come to renewal time. If you just add the intensity of red to dark brown, your hair is going to look very heavily coated, dull and very artificially red —like a woman with too much of the wrong shade of rouge on her face. Consider the brown factor when you're lightening to red, and soften its effect with gold.

All red hair—whether natural or chosen—fades faster than other colors. Therefore it is necessary to renew the color a bit more often to keep it fresh looking, sometimes with a rinse, even though it may not yet have grown out.

When redheads begin to gray, warm browns (such as red- and gold-browns) should be used in the red formula. This is because the gray (actually white) hairs are totally colorless and, without the warm brown formula, would take an almost pink-red cast and be wholly artificial looking.

RED Q'S AND A'S

What causes red-tinted hair to turn brassy orange?

Several factors could cause this: harsh shampoos, heated rollers used for settings too often, chemically treated pool water, harsh hair sprays, salt water deposits, air pollution or excessive exposure to the sun.

Can naturally red hair become paler with the use of just a lightener?

Usually not, since natural red is resistant to lightening and the results could be a brassy, unattractive red.

Can a brunette become a redhead simply by applying a lightener?

In the lightening process, dark brunette hair goes through a bright orange-red shade, a color that is hardly wearable. Color changes in the process of lightening are predictable and at some stage all hair develops red tones. Usually a toner is recommended after the lightening to keep the hair a soft, natural red, but most of the single-application reds lighten as well as color.

How can the most natural-looking red, with light and dark shades as well as highlights, be achieved?

When possible, the technique should be done by a highly-skilled colorist who has an artist's eye for the nuances of shading. The hair is sectioned into strands to be colored in the lighter and darker shades. The two or three tones must be applied very carefully to blend, with no contrasting lines of demarcation. The most natural-looking hair is done this way: the hair is first lightened and then subtly toned in two or three closely related shades, with the lightest at the front and side hairlines, the middle shade at the crown and on the ends, and the darkest in the back, at the nape—just as hair grows naturally on most heads. Obviously, this is not an easy, do-it-yourself operation.

How can you determine the most becoming shade of red?

Study your complexion. The very palest is best complemented by the lighter reds—all the way from strawberry blonde to the bright, brilliant, almost carrot-color with golden highlights. Skin that is so-called medium fair or creamy ivory goes well with the copper to deep auburn tones. Olive-toned complexions, dark skins and too-ruddy skins actually fight with red hair. When in doubt as to what looks best, try on wigs in various shades of red and, if you don't trust your own judgment, get a trusted hairdresser's appraisal. Be sure, however, to try on the wigs in a natural light. Artificial light (especially fluorescent) tends to minimize the red; hence you do not see the real picture.

36

What about henna, which seems to be having a revival?

Henna is a very old-fashioned—even ancient, as noted—hair-coloring agent. In the hands of an amateur, it can cause dryness or other damage with repeated use. Henna actually coats the hair; it fades more rapidly than other agents; it is more readily discolored by permanent waving or straightening; and it can kill the hair's natural highlights. Results are frequently inconsistent from application to application and the henna frequently is distributed unevenly on the hair shaft. With all the satisfactory red tints and rinses available, it is a "second best." I personally don't recommend it, as there are too many inconsistencies and unnatural effects.

Why doesn't hair turn out exactly the color shown on a product's color chart—especially the red colors?

First of all, when you look at your own hair color you are seeing the hair with light around and through it. When you look at the color chart you are looking at opaque inks on paper, without any see-through effect. Therefore, the charts can only be a close approximation. Finally, each individual's hair is as uniquely his or hers as fingerprints, and no two heads of hair will react exactly the same way to coloring. Things such as permanent waving and spraying extremely fine or coarse hair can change the outcome, too.

Will a temporary rinse produce those clear, lovely red lights?

Temporary rinses do not penetrate the hair shaft; they simply coat the hair. Repeated use of these will pile up the coating and ultimately make the hair look dull and lusterless. Semipermanent refresheners for faded red hair bring back some of the original luster.

What causes the purple or eggplant tones in hair that has been tinted with one of the red shades?

Darker red shades can produce those unwanted, shaded pur- 37

5. Janet is just fifteen. Her muddy-blonde hair lacked highlights. First step: conditioning, then cutting and shaping. Finally, with a prepackaged drugstore kit, or in the salon, a few strands around her face are lightened for a new soft, outdoorsy look with sunny highlights and sparkle and shine. (Photo by James Houghton, courtesy Clairol)

6. Mary Ann is twenty, just out of school and beginning her career. She was a blonde beginning to go brown, but feeling at heart a blonde. She wants to wear her hair medium long but maintain a look of professionalism at her job. Her hair needed toning, was brought to a pale yellow then given a slight wash of color to produce a soft, golden blonde—sunny and shining. The hair may be done with a prepackaged kit of pale blonde, working the color through the entire head for only three to five minutes. (Photo by James Houghton, courtesy Clairol)

7. Marilyn is in her mid-thirties and has drab brown hair, heavy in texture and too heavy-looking for her features. With a shampoo-in color, left on approximately twenty-five minutes, her hair is lightened to a golden brown. A few more pale golden highlights are added around her face for a softer look and to add reflection and light to her once very, very heavy-looking hair. (Photo by James Houghton, courtesy Clairol)

8.Cheri is thirty and was a blonde who used to highlight her hair but found it not glamorous enough. Now she is a double-process blonde: the whole head gently prelighted (the first time in the salon to be sure the right shade is achieved). A blonde shade was selected on the basis of skin tone, and since Cheri is brown-eyed, she is best as a light blonde with warm earthy tones. The cut and shaping of her shoulder-length hair allows for more versatility in styling; the color can look both glamorous at night and outdoorsy by day. (Photo by James Houghton, courtesy Clairol)

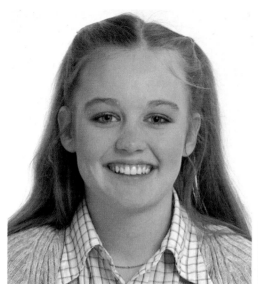
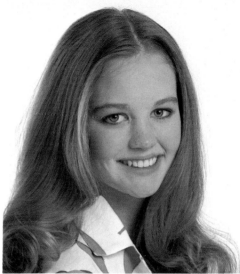
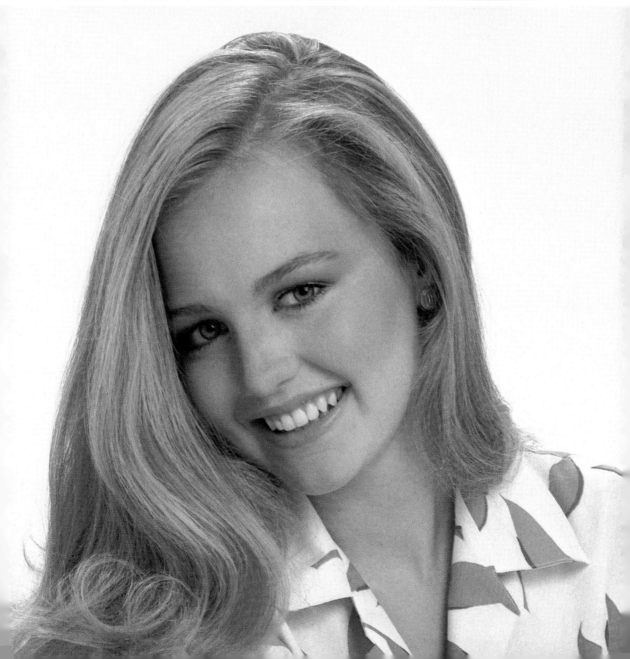

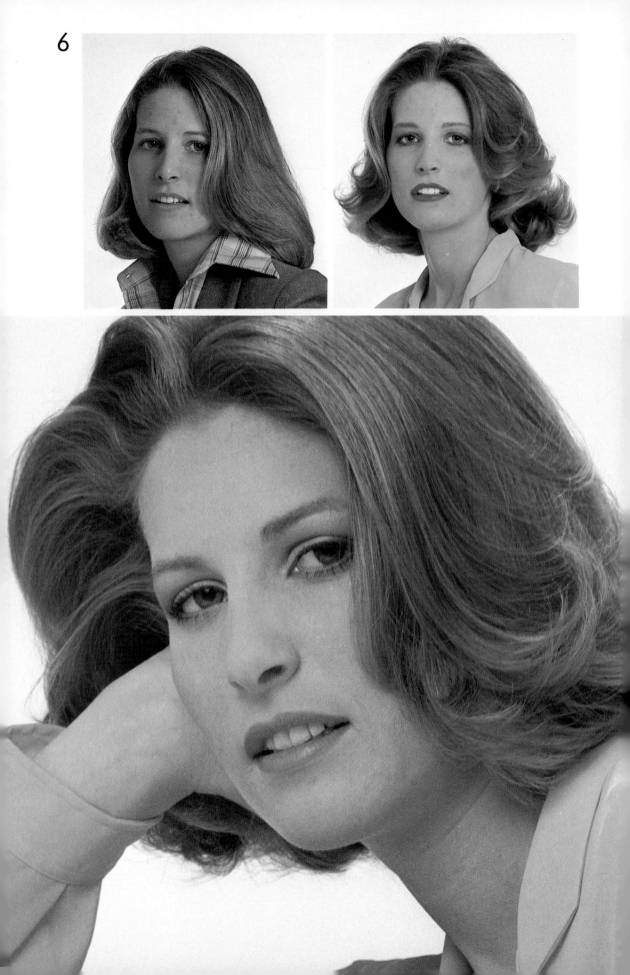

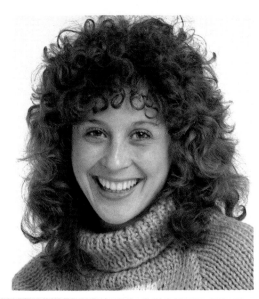

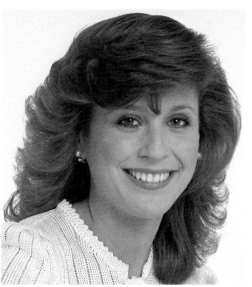

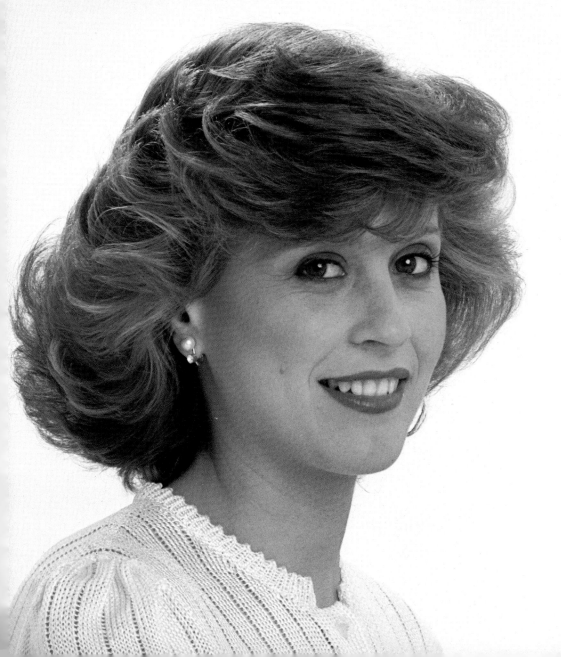

8

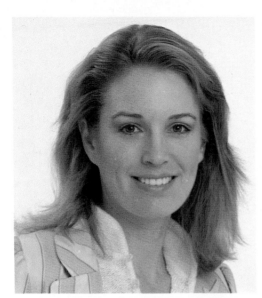
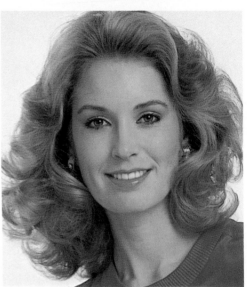
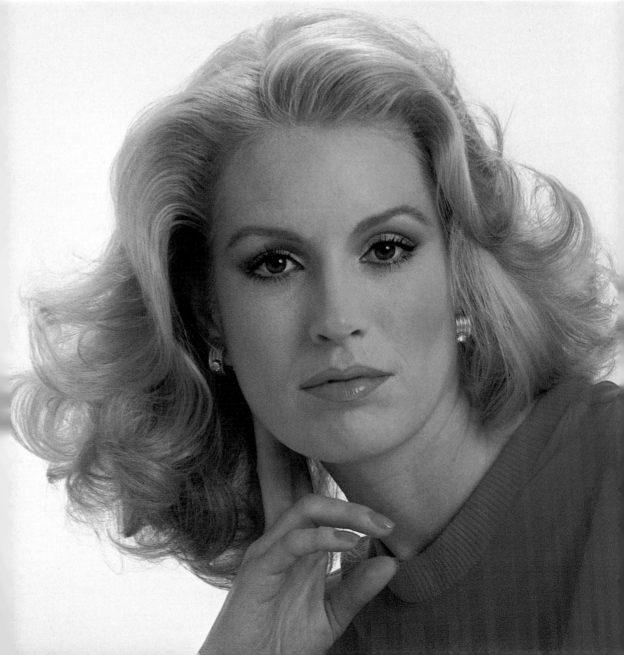

ples, especially if you have more than 15 percent gray hair. Another shade, one with more gold in it, should be selected. Alternatively, a small amount of gold tint (one part to three) added to the tint that produced the purple tone might do the trick of eliminating it. This, too, is difficult and should be left to the professional colorist in order to achieve the precise color that will compliment you the most. However, if it is done at home, be sure to discard all opened bottles after using part of the contents. Never use leftovers.

FASHION AND BEAUTY CUES

If red hair is becoming to you, you can probably be the most exciting woman in town. More than one redhead has asserted, "Not blondes, but redheads have more fun." Of course, it must be the right red for you and you must feel comfortable with red hair. You must live up to it—in your choice of makeup, in your fashions and in your hairstyle.

Red hair in general is so exciting as a color that it should really be styled in an understated way. It is at its best when worn very, very simply, smooth and soft. Never adopt trendy or gimmicky styles, because they will elicit those noted childhood nicknames. Avoid tight frizzles and chop-and-layer cuts. The softer and simpler the hairstyle, the more beautiful it is, because the color itself is so vibrant. When a lot of detail is added to the styling, red hair can become overpowering.

Colors that are very flattering in the redhead's wardrobe are the earth tones—the browns, beiges, russets—and anything warm and sunny. Certain shades of green—celadon and pale apple green—as well as camels and dove grays, enhance the appeal of red hair. Pale pink can be absolutely devastating on some redheads. Yellow is striking, too, but never the greenish yellows.

For the redhead's makeup, the spectrum is wide. Think gold and rich, warm browns. Soft, blushy pinks are good with the paler shades of red. Earth-tone shadows, blushers and lip colors complement the darker reds. Always keep in mind what's going on in the fashion world.

RED DO'S AND DON'TS

Do keep the flame bright. Red hair needs more watchfulness to keep its luster and brilliance. Use the gentlest shampoo—one that lubricates as it cleanses, without removing natural oils. Use lots of conditioners when hair tends to dryness. All toned and lightened hair needs regular conditioning. Even your cream conditioner, as well as shampoos, should be formulated for tinted hair.

DON'T expose red hair to unkind elements: drying winds, color-damaging strong sun, frizz-making dampness and rain. There are many conditioners with sun-screening agents that will help a great deal.

Do keep a wardrobe of scarves and cover-ups for wet weather, plus straw hats for shielding your bright locks from the sun. Remember to use only cotton scarves so that your hair can "breathe."

DON'T opt for red hair if your skin is too dark, and don't try to achieve a deep tan if you're a redhead. A tan is totally unbecoming to red hair. Besides, natural redheads are prone to freckles and redheads-by-choice tend to find that their hair color fades when exposed to strong sunlight for prolonged periods.

Do wait a week after having a permanent or a hair straightening before embarking on a new color.

DON'T use heat curlers and extremely hot blowers on freshly tinted red hair. Don't sit under hot dryers; instead, choose a warm temperature for hair settings.

6

Color You Brownette

Brown is the most common of all natural hair colors, and those who have it are lucky, since it can be changed, enhanced and varied more than any color in the hair spectrum.

"Jeannie with the light brown hair" wasn't celebrated in song without reason, for brown is the hair color of a thousand delights and hundreds of hues. More than likely *you* are a brownette, because more people have brown hair, by nature, than any other color. The brownette is not a brunette, with very dark brown or black hair. Neither is she a blonde, though she may have her light brown hair made lighter still and become a blonde—depending on her skin tones. On the other hand, she may, again depending on the compatibility of her complexion, opt for going brunette or red-haired. Her choices are limitless, because among the strands in her hair is every color nature ever conceived—from pale blonde and gold to red to almost black. She has but to decide which of these many colors she wishes to bring out to look her most attractive. There is literally no excuse for a brownette to have drab, mousy hair.

41

Just who is a brownette? She is too dark to be a blonde, though she may think of herself as a blonde because her hair was blonde during her childhood and gradually darkened. She is too light to be a brunette and not red enough to be a redhead. There are pale brownettes with fair skin (often prone to freckle), who usually have blue, blue-green or gray eyes. There are warm brown brownettes with creamy skin that tans to a golden hue and eyes that are brown, hazel, or sometimes blue or green. Then there are darker brownettes with olive skin and, usually, brown eyes (though they are sometimes hazel or gray-green). The dark brownette borders on being a brunette, but her hair frequently has so many red and gold highlights that it appears much lighter, especially after it has been freshly shampooed and often after long exposure to strong sunlight.

Since our world is largely composed of brownettes, it is small wonder that so many hair-coloring products are devoted to enhancing—or even changing—that very special category of hair color. "Perk up the brownette" seems to be the message. Make minks out of mice! There are shades that do not so much change nature as make the most of it. There are shades to deepen or lighten, shades to blot out gray or white (nothing makes a brownette look duller than a mix of non-color throughout her hair), shades that bring out the gold or the red inherent in the brownette, and shades that simply add sparkle to the natural hair. These are formulated in rinses—temporary to rinse in and rinse out, or semipermanent that fades away gradually and won't rub off, lasting for several weeks. These are convenient and easy to use—both at home and in the salon —and offer the widest latitude for experiment without the commitment of permanent hair coloring. Once a brownette has decided on her favorite look and color, permanent colorings may be applied at home or in the salon—again, not to change the basic brownette coloring, but to add sparkle and play it up. These products contain special conditioners to add new sheen and highlights along with the color. As noted, the brownette has the widest choice of color within her spectrum than any other hair shade. She can go gradually, subtly, from the color she was born with to very, very light or very, very dark, easily and attractively.

Part of being an attractive brownette is a matter of attitude. To be one, one must *want* to have brown hair. After all, brownettes are in the best of company in the world of beautiful women. Just look at the range of shining brown hair—the company you can keep—among such as Princess Caroline, First Lady of the United States Nancy Reagan, Sally Field, one-time Miss America Phyllis George Brown, Mary Tyler Moore, Brooke Shields, Elizabeth Ashley, Ali McGraw, Diane Keaton, and scores more, including always at least one brownette playing in *Charlie's Angels*.

No, you just can't sit there with your brown hair and moan over the fact that you're not a ravishing redhead, a siren blonde or a smoldering brunette. There's literally gold in those strands and it's up to you to bring it out and wake it up to a super-glorious head of hair that turns heads because of its special radiance. No other color lends itself so delightfully to special effects (see Chapter 9), to highlighting and to the dozens of nuances of pretty, shining hair color.

During the brownette's youngest years, playing up the softness of color and keeping the hair lustrous in a regular program of maintenance is generally all that's necessary, but the regimen must be strictly adhered to. Regular shampooing and conditioning are musts. If the hair tends to be oily and to look stringy two days after it has been shampooed, then shampoo it every day and choose a shampoo formulated for oily hair. Brush it before shampooing, to loosen the scalp and distribute the oil throughout the hair. Don't be afraid to wash the hair every day; there is no such thing as too much cleanliness. If the hair has been overexposed to the sun, chances are the ends are faded, dry, even split. Have hair trimmed of the damaged areas and give it a good conditioning treatment before shampooing. Even if the hair is worn long, the ends should be periodically trimmed, if only a quarter of an inch, to make it more manageable and to get rid of (and prevent additional) splits and dried ends.

During the twenties and thirties, brownettes will enjoy experimenting with highlighting rinses to perk up hair that seems to be going dull and lifeless. From thirty to forty, when gray or white strands begin to show, all-over color to cover the gray and brighten the hair is recommended. This is especially true when the hair is 20 percent to 30 percent gray; the color treatment will make the hair more manageable and give the no-color strands better texture. In very dark brunettes, gray streaks and strands—a silver fox look, perhaps—can be attractive, but the lighter or brownette hair simply loses its radiance, since there isn't enough contrast in the strands.

After fifty, the brownette should look to the lighter, more golden shades, or even some of the subtle red hues. Never should she go dark brunette or black, no matter what her skin tones are, since very dark shades simply emphasize aging lines.

The goal of all brownettes is to capitalize on the varied hues found in their hair. Constant conditioning is not only a sparkle-maker but a preventive measure against flat, dull brown hair. While the latitude for color change is broad, adding light or dark shades should be done gradually, carefully, subtly, in order not to mask the inherent loveliness of brown hair, with its myriad lights and shadows.

BROWNETTE Q'S AND A'S

How can brown-tinted hair be kept from turning red a few weeks after it has been colored?

Your natural hair probably has a lot of red in it and, if you prefer not to accentuate this, you should change your hair-coloring formula. Choose an ash-brown shade instead. If this doesn't solve the problem, then you might try a drabbing rinse to modify the red/gold tones. Choose one formulated for gray or white hair with a name such as "silver," "slate," "smoke," or "white."

What causes the ends of hair that has been colored light brown for a number of years to get darker than the rest of the hair, and how can this be corrected?

The hair ends are always the dryest part of any head of hair; therefore, they are porous and over-receptive to color during the tinting process. The same over-porous ends are probably split and subject to breakage. The easiest solution, of course, is to have the ends periodically trimmed. However, if this isn't desired and long hair is preferred, follow one of these procedures during the next tinting session. You can coat the ends with a conditioner before applying color, then bring the color over the conditioner. Another method is to wait until the last five minutes of the process to tint the ends; dilute some of the tint with water for application to the ends only.

Is there any temporary touch-up for gray or white regrowth around the hairline of light-brown tinted hair?

Yes. There are color crayons for this purpose, but these often make the hair feel sticky or greasy. A good way is simply to use a matching brown mascara wand and lightly apply color to the offending regrowth.

Would the tendrils of brown hair at the temples and nape of an updo look attractive if lightened? If so, how light should they be?

By nature, hair around the face is lighter and that at the nape is darker. Face tendrils can be attractive when lightened about two shades. At the nape, however, it is more natural looking to lighten the tendrils only one shade—just to achieve a slightly lighter brown than the rest of the hair.

*Can a brownette successfully have her hair streaked with
very pale blonde?*

Only if the streaks are subtly, carefully done so as not to
look like stripes. The shade of brownette must be taken into
consideration, and the strands to be lightened must be carefully
selected—more near the face, where hair is naturally lighter,
and less at the crown and back, where hair is normally darker.
The lighter brown the hair is, the paler the streaks can be.
There always should be a subtle blending, never a harsh,
defined contrast.

*If hair is lightened just around the face and the rest of the
naturally brown hair is not tinted, will retouching be necessary
very often?*

If the hair is lightened from roots to ends, it will need retouching as often as if the entire head of hair were lightened—
about every four to five weeks, depending on the speed of hair
growth. The lightening of areas of the hair on very light
brown hair will not be so obvious as on darker hair, so retouching time may often be extended. In any case, however,
once any or all of the hair is lightened it must be protected
with special shampoos, conditioners, and hair sprays formulated
for tinted hair.

*What can be done to brown hair that has been streaked, if
the streaks turned out too gold/yellow?*

Rinse all of the hair with a drabber to tone down the gold,
or tint the hair all over in a darker, warmer brown until the
streaks grow out.

*How can one get a sunstreaked look on brown hair without
constantly sunbathing?*

This effect is achieved by lightening selected strands of hair
around the face with a creamy lightener that has a built-in
conditioner, then using a blonde toner in the preferred shade.

Also, if you are graying, an all-over sunkissed look can be achieved by using a blonde-highlighting temporary or semipermanent color two shades lighter than the natural color of the hair. These are fortified with conditioners and can simply be shampooed in.

Should "in-between" brown hair—neither very light nor dark, but just a dull "medium"—be tinted lighter or darker?

The "in-between" brownette can go either way, lighter or darker; what dictates which is more attractive is the wearer's complexion and eye coloring. Darker skins and darker eyes usually look better with darker hair. The fair-skinned brownette can go either way. There are really no hard-and-fast rules; it is a matter of deciding which looks best on any given individual. Trying temporary rinses—those that shampoo in and shampoo out with ease—is one way to determine what is most becoming. Trying on wigs in various shades of brown, blonde and brunette, even red, also can be helpful in making a decision.

What about wigs? Can they be colored to match your new hair color?

The hair on wigs can be tinted, stripped, bleached and dyed in many ways. A good wig, however—of human hair, hand-sewn into a well-fitting foundation—is usually costly and should be cleaned, recolored and restyled only by a professional.

Can two or three shades of brown or gold or red be used on a brownette for a tone-on-tone effect?

Tone-on-tone coloring is tricky and difficult to do at home. To use three shades takes great skill. The brownette, as noted, has many different-colored strands throughout the hair and tinting it is often just a matter of accentuating those preferred colors—for instance, the warm reds or the golds. Today's hair

47

colorings are formulated not only to lighten or darken, but to brighten, condition and bring out previously unnoticed highlights. If you are a dark brownette, you may well get the effect you're hunting for simply by going two shades lighter with a single, all-over application of color.

How long will the blonde tips last on brownette hair? Does it need retouching often?

Since tipping is usually done on short hair and since the process involves only the ends of the hair, not the roots, retouching is not necessary. The tipping will last until it is cut off. This probably will be in about four haircuts, depending on how quickly the hair grows.

Can a sixty-year-old brownette successfully become a very dark brunette?

Almost never. Very dark shades of hair are extremely unflattering to aging skins; they accentuate facial lines and wrinkles. The rare exceptions are fair-skinned people whose complexions have remained clear and unlined.

BROWNETTE DO'S AND DON'TS

Do make a patch test at least twenty-four hours before coloring your hair for the first time or when you change brands of coloring products. Make one also if, after coloring several times, any sensitivity is noticed.

Don't color your hair if your scalp is abraded, has any sores or cuts or shows symptoms of any scalp disease.

Do make a preliminary strand test before applying tints or lighteners. Make strand tests several times as color develops or lightening action progresses.

Don't save unused tints that have been mixed by you with lightening agents.

Do store partly used, unmixed coloring products with a tightly screwed-on cap and in a cool, dark place.

Don't lighten or tint hair immediately after a permanent or hair-relaxing treatment. Wait at least a week, if possible, after conditioning.

Do make a record of the time it takes for your hair to reach the proper shade when using coloring.

Don't prepare coloring or lightening mixtures ahead of time. Apply them at once after mixing them, and follow the manufacturer's directions *exactly*.

Do be sure to check expiration dates on the packages of hair-coloring products, and don't use outdated ones.

Don't try to match a shade from a color chart when your own hair is soiled or wet. The match will prove to be inaccurate, since hair in that condition is always darker.

Do work with proper light when coloring brownette—or any other color—hair. Best is daylight directed from the north. Next best is incandescent light. Least desirable is fluorescent light, which gives the hair a false bluish color and masks the reds and golds so that accurate results cannot be obtained.

Don't ever permit coloring and lightening solutions to get near the eyes. Coat the eye area and lids with petroleum jelly or cold cream before coloring or lightening. If eyes are accidentally splashed, immediately flush them with clear water for several minutes to remove all traces of the mixtures.

Do be sure to remove all rinses, coatings, henna compounds and other products from the hair before attempting to apply new tints and lighteners. If necessary, have a deep conditioning treatment to cleanse the hair first. Then wait several days before tinting or lightening, until the hair is slightly soiled and natural oils have again been dispersed through the hair. It is preferable not to tint or lighten on freshly shampooed hair.

DON'T let too much time elapse between retouchings if brownette hair has been lightened. When you begin to see root show-through, other people can see it even more in bright sunlight.

BROWNETTE FASHION AND BEAUTY CUES

Just as brownette hair has the broadest spectrum of tints and tones from which to choose hair coloring, so, too, do brownettes have the widest selection of makeup and fashion colors at their disposal. If you stay within your category as a brownette, all the warmer colors can be yours to complement your hair. The coral tones, soft oranges, beiges, and a blending of camels and grays, sometimes called "greige," are the most flattering. In other words, choose colors that have yellow, orange and earth tones in them—all soft and subtle—so that the vibrancy and light-reflecting properties of your hair are enhanced.

The muted lipsticks and blushers are much more flattering to the brownette, as opposed to the dark brunette who looks best with clear, almost primary colors for eyes, lips and cheeks. For the brownette, the warm, earthy shades, hints of bronze, honey, peach and muted pastels do the trick most effectively. The same earth tones in fashion give her an aura of elegance. Stark black clothing doesn't play up the inherent loveliness of golden brown or reddish brown hair the way ginger, warm beige and nutmeg-brown fabrics do. In summer, when the hair tends to be more golden, soft pastels and subtle clay colors are your best bet.

Eye makeup depends on eye color, of course, but again the brownette must go soft and subtle. Never use jet-black mascara or brow color, never harshly thick black liner. Touches of bronze gloss on lids or an iridescent topaz will play up flecks of gold in both hair and eye color. For the brownette whose eyes are more green than gray, a soft jade can be used for evening eye makeup. Gray is the most common eye color of the brownette; it is often a chameleon color, sometimes appearing blue, hazel or green. Any one of those shades can be emphasized with makeup, but always in the subtler shades, never in the clear, primary ones. The eye shadows should have warmth —brown with gold in it, beige with a bit of red in it, muted turquoise, or softened spice tones.

The outdoor brownette whose hair has a perennial sun-kissed look can opt for fashions in sunny shades—coral, yellows, tawny tones. The more fragile brownette with pale skin looks best in soft pastels. Bright reds, shocking pinks and vibrant greens and blues can only kill the subtleties of the brownette and should, in almost every case, be left to the realm of the dark brunette. Even stark white isn't advisable, but a creamy off-white can be infinitely complimentary.

7

Color You Brunette

Dark brown, almost black, hair is the true brunette. Dazzling on the young, dramatic in the middle years if the complexion is clear and flawless, it must never be allowed to go matte and flat, nor patent-leathery.

While the witch in the fairy tale and the siren of fiction are always raven tressed, the fact is that some of the most exciting beauties in the world are brunettes. (Do you wonder which color I favor? The color I prefer is the one that makes you look and feel the most beautiful.) Numbered among the most celebrated brunettes are Jacqueline Onassis, Elizabeth Taylor, Gina Lollobrigida, Ava Gardner, Jane Russell, Claudia Cardinale, Sophia Loren, Jaclyn Smith, Helen Gurley Brown, Anna Moffo Sarnoff, and Hedy Lamarr in her day. All have dark hair, ranging from deep brown with gold and reddish highlights to nearly blue-black. There are, in fact, almost as many shades of brunette as there are brunettes. She who has very dark hair must have a fine sense of fashion and cosmetics to live up to it, for it is one of the most difficult colors to wear.

Despite the myriad variations of the brunette category, it may be divided roughly according to skin and eye color and even personality. There is the sultry brunette, with hair close to jet black, skin on the olive side and dark, almost smoldering, eyes. Then there is the creamy-to-fair-skinned dark brunette with vivid blue eyes—often an Irish woman with some Spanish ancestry. Not so dark, with hair more brown than black and showing a hint of red, is the brunette whose complexion has a tawny glow. She may sport freckles in some cases, and her eyes may be brown, hazel, green or blue. Finally, there is the very dark, more-black-than-brown brunette, whose skin may range from fair to a forever-tan shade and whose eyes may be almost any of the range of colors.

Whatever type of brunette you are, remember that, because of its dark mass, your hair attracts the eye, so its shape and condition are always on view. Its silhouette—your hairdo—is most important; it is a bold frame for the face and the eyes. Not only your face shape, but your neck, your height and your figure must be taken into consideration when you or your hairdresser select a style to compliment the whole of you.

Very dark hair is most attractive on the very young—or the youthful. As one ages, too-dark hair is harsh and unkind to fading complexions and serves only to emphasize lines and wrinkles in the skin. The rule is to go lighter rather than darker with time, softening the color just a little, lightening and warming, even adding a few shadings or highlights to give the hair luster and sheen. Dark hair *must* shine, must be conditioned to sparkle. If it doesn't, it will have a dull, dry, matte look. Very dark hair absorbs rather than reflects light, so it needs all the light it can get, on its own or with color and conditioning assistance. It should never be colored totally black, or black with a definite blue cast, nor should it have a rusty, burnt look. If the brunette needs warmth to offset these problems, then her route should be toward a golden brown. The

9. Kate is also in her thirties. Her hair was red, became faded and lost its golden-copper lights. Her need: to be a positive redhead. A shampoo-in color in medium golden red does the basic trick for Kate. Added to this is the lightening of selected strands with a pale golden blonde to reflect light and add sparkle and shine. (Photo by James Houghton, courtesy Clairol)

10. Barbara's hair was the darkest of all the women here, too dark and too artificial-looking, making her face seem too tiny and giving her hair a heavy look. It is lightened to a medium-brown with a shampoo-in color—one part darkest ash blonde and two parts lightest brown. Highlights were also added around her face to soften her facial features and to reflect light. The result—a considerable lift and lightening of both hair and complexion for a more exciting overall appearance. (Photo by James Houghton, courtesy Clairol)

11. Evelyn is thirty-two, beginning to go gray, had a "tired" look. Her gray-brown hair was conditioned (gray hair is often dryer) for more bounce and vitality, then treated to a little lighter honey-blonde shade with pale golden highlights. She might even go in the direction of reddish blonde for an even more lively look. She was tired of people thinking she was older and while she loved and enjoyed her gray hair, she wanted to look more youthful. She should not go too dark or too blonde—either is more aging. Hair should be and is slightly shaded so that regrowth won't be quickly noticeable. With shaded hair, regrowth becomes just another dimension of color. (Photo by James Houghton, courtesy Clairol)

12. Color him, too. (Photo by Neal Barr, courtesy Clairol)

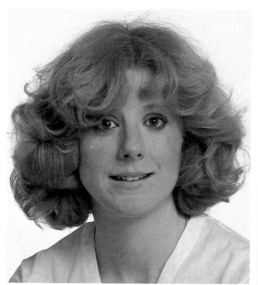

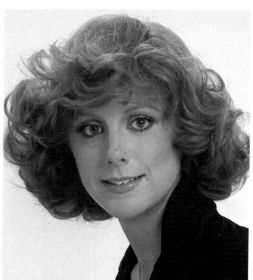

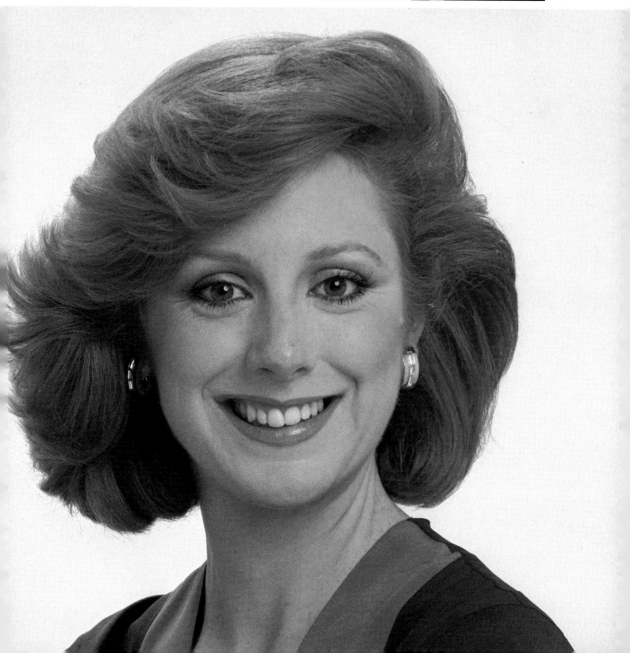

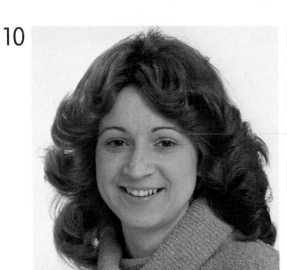
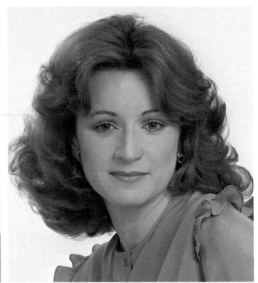
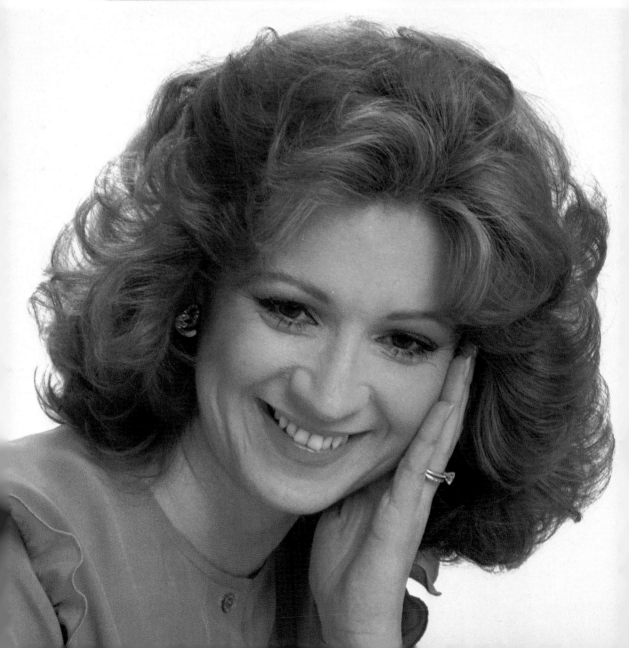

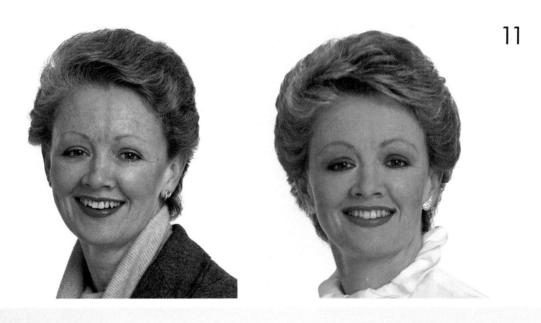

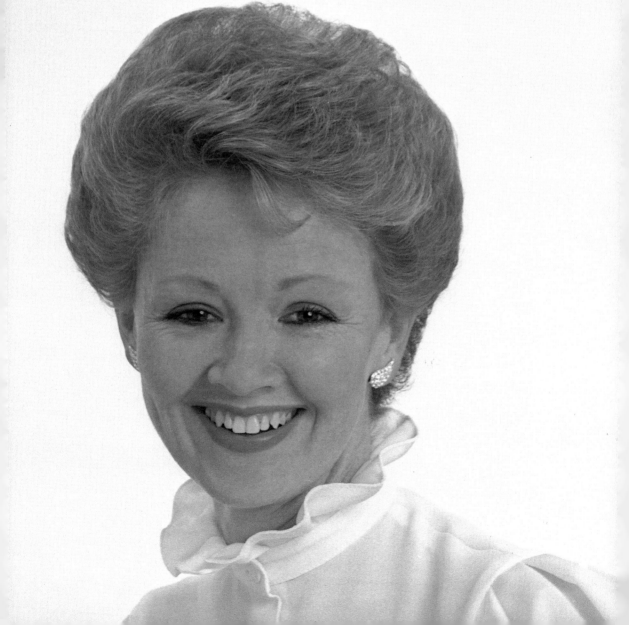

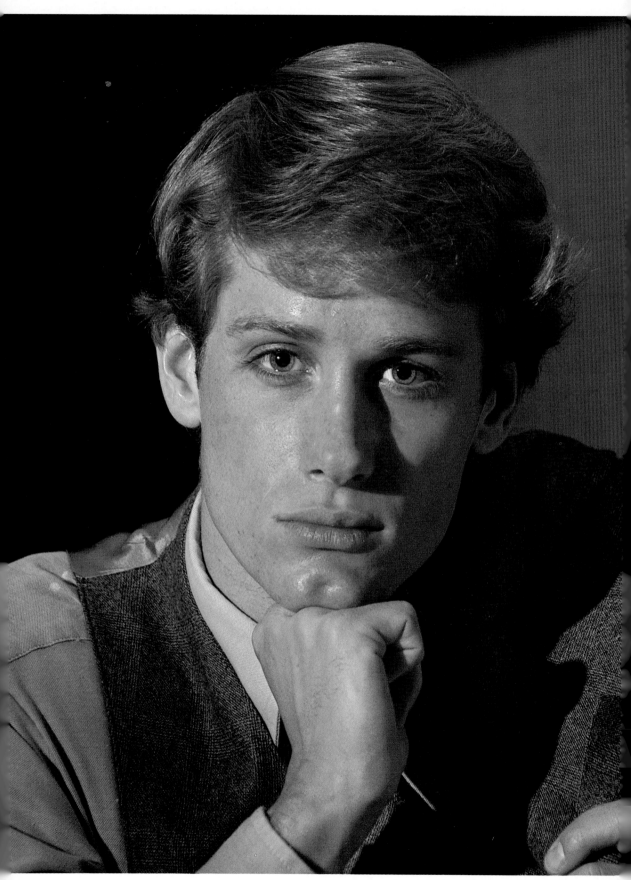

newest brunette colors are softer than ever before and are formulated to eliminate that rusty look.

Totally black hair exists naturally only among Oriental peoples and among certain primitive tribes. Most women who appear to have black hair under dim lights will, in fact, reveal much warmer brown tones, even hints of red, in the sun or under bright lights. For them, as they begin to age, very little added color is necessary—just enough, and gradually, to enrich the hair so that it doesn't look washed out, like a photograph that's begun to fade.

The time to begin taking stock of color is generally at thirty. A touch of softness and warmth—the merest touch of color—and dark hair can still be dramatic, still exciting. The hairstyle, too, should be softer, worn a little looser to encourage a play of light and shadow. By age thirty-nine the brunette usually should become more glowing, warmer, with the subtlest touch of gold flicking through the hair in a now-you-see-it-now-you-don't way. As time marches on, the same coloring treatment should be followed, probably more frequently and a little more intensely, until gray or white hair begins to take over. As the light fades from the face, instead of being a deep, strong brunette, one should become a softer, warmer one, with hair that reflects light on the skin and gives it a certain warm glow.

Exceptions to this—there are exceptions to every rule—are women who have a strong sense of identity, very positive personalities, and a highly developed personal style in their mature years. Examples are jet-black-haired, severely coiffed women like fashion arbiter Diana Vreeland and fashion designers Mary McFadden and Gloria Vanderbilt. Usually, they also wear non-colors—black or white—or vibrant reds and other primary colors. Their hairstyles and hair color accentuate the color impact with marked individuality. On the other end of the spectrum, there are also exceptions to the rule. Basically brunette Sophia Loren goes softer with warm red tones; Raquel Welch and Barbara Walters attractively opt for soft glints of gold, with the latter becoming almost a golden brownette, which in my opinion is much more beautiful and softer.

During the youthful years, maintenance of brunette hair is relatively easy because it is just a matter of retaining and intensifying the color, while highlighting it. When a brunette begins to be more than 20 percent gray, though, she needs, in most cases, to use a more permanent type of coloring, which will hold because it penetrates the hair shaft and cannot be washed out. The problem with gray hair in a brunette is not only that it is more obvious by virtue of contrast, but the texture of the gray is often very different—coarser, even corkscrew-curly. Permanent hair coloring, then, with its built-in conditioning elements, will make the hair more uniform in texture and more manageable.

On the other hand, brunettes of a very dark hue have an advantage over their fair-haired friends by the very nature of the contrast. A natural streak can be a dramatic asset. So-called pepper-and-salt hair on a youthful face can be attractive. If the gray or white hairs serve only to dull the hair, though, it's wiser to cover them with carefully selected color.

Whether you do or don't color your brunette hair, be scrupulous about its condition. Keep it glossy and vital. If it's dry and unmanageable, condition it, but avoid those after-shampoo cream rinses that leave a dulling film on the hair. Keep your scalp loose by massaging as you shampoo. Take remedial steps instantly if dandruff appears or even if your scalp is so dry that it flakes. Get help from a dermatologist if the situation persists. This applies to all types of hair, but little white flakes are certainly most painfully obvious on brunettes.

Remember, think brunette. In a way, being one requires you to live up to the very positive and dramatic qualities of dark hair. A shy brunette is a contradiction in imagery.

BRUNETTE Q'S AND A'S

Can a very dark brunette go blonde?

If you're a dark brunette, don't even think blonde. Only a rare few have crossed that bridge with success, and even they find maintenance, combatting regrowth, and recoloring a constant, tedious problem. For most brunettes, light blonde hair will be incompatible with their skin tones, making makeup a matter of great artistry. For the busy woman of today, all of this is too time-consuming. Additionally, unless this step is taken with the aid of a highly skilled colorist, the risk of breakage on some textures of brunette hair is high during the decolorization process.

Are there special shampoos for brunettes?

Just as for other hair colors, the texture and condition of the hair dictate the shampoo. For finer, thinner hair, choose a delicate shampoo. Thicker and stronger hair can be treated to less gentle cleansers. If the hair is either very oily or very dry, shampoos formulated for those conditions should be used. In either case, in the salon or at home, never use hot water to wash or rinse the hair, and avoid very hot dryers, especially after freshly coloring your hair.

What can be done between colorings about roots showing?

Even slight growth around the hairline on hair that is colored brunette becomes quickly visible. A marvelous tip: Between colorings, blend in the regrowth at the hairline with mascara carefully brushed on when the hair is almost dry after shampooing. Finish grooming, brushing and arranging the hair; the mascara will blend in nicely. Wax crayons, which are commonly used for the purpose, are not nearly as effective, because the wax gets into the scalp and gives a sticky look to the hair.

Can one successfully put gray streaks in the hair?

A streak or two, which sometimes appear in nature, can be

dramatic, especially on very dark hair, but they usually look very unnatural. If highlights are to be put into the hair, it is best done by a skilled colorist. Highlights should be carefully placed and should be done subtly, without too much contrast, or they will look artificial. Leaving out strands of the gray hair to suggest streaks when the brunette colors her hair usually looks very unnatural and generally is not successful.

Why does brunette hair turn reddish in the sun, especially after vacations at the beach?

Excessive exposure to sun can really fade dark brunette hair. That and the added insult of too much salt water drying the hair can do it. Always rinse the hair after swimming, even if only with cool, clear water. The sun damage may require a slight color boost—very little, just to enrich the hair after a good conditioning treatment and a trimming of the dried ends.

Should a brunette with Elizabeth Taylor's coloring go lighter or darker as she ages and gray appears?

With Miss Taylor's striking violet eyes and very white skin, the most attractive color treatment would be blending down the white hair to make it look smokier. This would soften the look, yet keep the hair dramatic against the lovely skin tone. Who in the world could be compared with Elizabeth Taylor, though? There is only one.

If a dark brunette with nearly black hair wanted to be blonde, what would be the procedure?

First, all pigment would have to be removed before any tones or shades of blonde could be introduced. This is such an extremely radical step that it is not usually recommended. It is almost like putting a piece of fabric, black or dark brown, in strong laundry bleach and trying to make it white; the time it would take would so damage the fibers that there would be almost nothing left of the fabric.

What about going from brunette to auburn?

If one is a warm, not a cool, brunette, this can be very attractive—but a very dark auburn with a reddish cast depends
on the skin tone. If one has a lot of yellow or pink in the skin,
a reddish color is not advisable. The fair—almost white-
skinned—can wear almost any color, but the best rule is to
take into consideration that after a certain age a rich auburn or
sunny brown can be much more youthful looking.

What kinds of conditioners are best for brunette hair?

Very light conditioners, which do not leave a film on the
hair and give an oily look, are preferable. It is important that
dark hair not have a greasy look. Almost all conditioners
should be rinsed out after use, with the exception of a revitalizing lotion, which gives the hair a silky and shiny look.

*What can one do about stains around the hairline and on fa-
cial skin when color is applied?*

Protect your skin with a very light, easily removable cream
or petroleum jelly—around the hairline, behind the ears—and,
if you're doing the coloring, your entire face. Some skins are
almost like sponges, and dark colors especially adhere to those.

*How can dark coloring stains best be removed from the skin
or scalp while coloring the hair?*

Take a strand of the hair where tint has been applied, wipe
off the tint and rub the strand on the spot. The color will lift
off the skin and adhere to the strand. Another way is to take
the corner of a damp terry-cloth towel and rub it off.

*Sometimes the color rinse used on very dark hair comes off
on combs, brushes and pillowcases. Why?*

Either a poor quality rinse is being used too often, or the
color rinse has not been applied correctly and has not been
thoroughly rinsed with clear tepid water afterward. The pile-

up of coating thus rubs off on whatever it comes in contact with.

How can spatters of dark color be removed from porcelain sinks and tile floors?

With any good bleach-action cleanser. Spatterers might find it easier to use foamy shampoo colors rather than liquid ones, thereby eliminating drips and splatters.

Is there any red in nearly black hair? Why does black-tinted hair begin to have a reddish, rusty cast between colorings?

Even the darkest hair has some red in it. Strong light and long exposure to intense sunlight often make it show up, especially as the natural color fades with age. Tinted black may lose its intensity between colorings if a too-strong shampoo is used—one that strips the color. Always use a gentle to delicate shampoo for color-treated hair. Clean hair always makes the brunette sparkle.

BRUNETTE FASHION AND BEAUTY CUES

Very dark hair—truly brunette—is a dramatic focal point that dictates a clear-cut approach to fashion and makeup. Whether you're the breezy outdoor type, the vibrant Irish gamine, or the *femme fatale* indoor brunette, there can be no in-between or haphazard approach to color, line and design in fashion, and no timidity in the use of makeup. For you the words are "clear," "vibrant," "vivid."

The colors that are most flattering on the brunette are those with very little softness and warmth: strong, clear blues, vivid pinks, violets, bold reds. Stark white and black are dramatic non-colors which also underscore the dark mass of hair that makes a brunette stand out. No muddy taupes, olives or muted colors should be chosen by the brunette. Simple, pure-line fashion designs heighten the drama for most, except for the rare, fragile Scarlett O'Hara type with flawless, nearly white skin. For her, the frills and flounces, in moderation, can be an interesting counterplay.

Makeup is all-important. For the most part, it should be a little stronger, more vivid, than for the other types in the hair-color spectrum. Strong, clear reds and pinks are best for the lips—none of the earthy, bronze or pastel shades. Orange- and yellow-tinged lip colors are to be avoided. Blushers must be clear; sallow skin and sallow colors are not complimentary to very dark hair. Focus should be on eye makeup, because eyes become even more important with the dark frame of hair. Faded or graying brows and lashes must be intensified with dark pencil and mascara so that the eyes don't wash out. Blue eyes are especially exciting on brunettes. If your eyesight is not acute and glasses are worn, you might consider colored contact lenses. Blue or gray, as well as dark brown or hazel eyes on brunettes can be enhanced and dramatized with careful use of liners—the darkest shades—and subtle use of blue, smoke or silvery eye shadow for special occasions. The shadow should be strongest near the upper lashes and gradually fade back over the lid until it is barely there. Never should it be obvious, but always a barely perceptible accent to enhance the natural eye color.

BRUNETTE DO'S AND DON'TS

DON'T choose to be a black-as-night brunette if your skin is so sallow or so olive-toned that makeup can't correct it. Go for a warmer, more golden brunette or one of the myriad brown shades.

DON'T postpone coloring sessions—three to four weeks is the longest span advisable for most people—so that visible roots destroy your dramatic brunette look.

DON'T wear a hairstyle that's so severe you look like a figure in an Art Deco poster—unless your skin is flawless and your features are perfect. Nearly black hair, more than any other color, emphasizes and underscores every feature fault on the human face.

Do be scrupulous about shampoos. Stringy, oily dark hair, by the very nature of its color, is more noticeable than all others.

Do go gradually, never in one giant step, to the darkest brunette if your hair is fading or if you've decided that brunette is the perfect color for you, your complexion, your eye color. An extreme change is more difficult to reverse in dark colors when you make the wrong decision and the color turns out to be unbecoming.

8

The Gray Illusion

White hair is becoming a rarity in today's world of undetectable coloring. It can be truly stunning when it is beautifully coiffed and meticulously maintained.

Just as the blue of the sky is an optical illusion, gray hair is not really gray, but white hair scattered throughout pigmented hair, which gives a look of gray. Until all or most of the hair loses its pigment, it may be referred to as "pepper-and-salt," "steel-gray" or "silver." The process is generally gradual and can begin as early as your teens or as late as your seventies. When all the melanin or pigment has gone from every hair, it is white—pure, platinum white. This occurs very late in life, unless there has been premature severe illness or stress, extreme diet deficiency, or hereditary factors that dictate such phenomena as pure white hair from birth, as in albinos.

The decision to go or stay "gray" or white is, of course, a purely personal one. When the first strands appear, many women see them as a sign of aging. True as that may be, there is no cause for alarm. The chapters in this book offer all the ways of concealment, but here we address those who prefer to keep every white strand and go gray or white with grace and pride. Surely everyone can call to mind at least one beautiful silvery head that complemented the wearer's complexion and eyes, while standing out dramatically in a crowd. There is a certain kindness in nature's way of lightening the hair as we grow older, since light and white give a certain lift to tired, aging skins and fading eyes. Usually the first white strands of hair appear around the face, where light is most needed. When the first strands appear in a dark brunette, the hair color may be termed "salt-and-pepper." As the unpigmented hair increases, it may be called "steel." The hair eventually progresses to silver and then the most glorious of all, shining white. It is the brunette who does this most elegantly because of the striking contrast of light and dark. Blonde and brown-haired women, on the other hand, until hair is totally white, must suffer through stages of drab, almost muddy color. Their hair sometimes turns yellowish in an unbecoming way. Redheads will look faded, washed out, with the warm gold tones gradually disappearing and the hair turning almost pinkish.

Silver hair can be glorious, but you cannot simply stand still and wait for it to happen. Your colorist will tell you when you can go gray or white. When you do, you'll need a new outlook on hair care, on the fashions you wear, on your makeup and your accessories. Money is not among the chief criteria in these matters; taste and intelligence are.

If you are in the enviable dark brunette category, you may let nature take its course, relying on conditioners and rinses to maintain healthy, glossy, beautiful hair. If you are very pale blonde, the white strands may make your hair look lighter and you will depend on gentle rinses and conditioners to add highlights to offset dullness. As more white appears, your colorist may advise toning the hair to add warmth to tide you over until all is silvery. Brownettes, dark blondes and redheads will want to follow the same program during their long wait, using permanent coloring until the hair is clearly and definitely all white.

There are rinses, shampoo tints and special-effects tones formulated specifically for gray or white hair. The highlighting, conditioner-fortified shades of gray range from steel, smoke, slate and other dark tones to such as platinum, pearl and silver. Some are shampoo-to-shampoo temporary highlighters, some are semipermanent (wearing off gradually after a month or two). They add a finish, rather like buffing fine silver and making a play of delicate light and shadow. They also take care of the bane of the light-gray-haired and the white-haired by eliminating the yellow that often tinges such hair.

Above all, the silver-haired should avoid fantasy colors. Those, too, are a thing of the past; the shocking blue- or even pink-toned rinses are unbecoming and unnatural. For those who opt for lovely white hair, the daily care should be intensified to offset dryness and coarseness of texture, with faithful and regular use of conditioners and extra-gentle, "for fine hair" shampoos. Only tepid water should be used throughout the cleansing process, and hair should be kept away from the extreme heat of electric curlers and too-hot dryers. Brushing should be done sparingly and with a soft, natural-bristle brush. Scalp massages—both during shampoos and in between—are advisable to keep the scalp loose, the circulation active, and the hair lively and bouncy.

Special attention should be paid to the coiffing of white hair. Long bobs and Trilby locks are not suitable for the mature woman. The hair is best cut short, since long-hair updos put too much strain on this fragile kind of hair. A close, softly wide-waved style, with a little fullness near the face, is a good bet. For the curly-haired, a short-short, all-over open-curl look is frequently attractive. Never wear white or gray hair in a straight, severe boy-cut. Also avoid hairdos with long downward lines, which emphasize deepening facial lines around the mouth and the eyes.

Choose soft, pale eye makeup and lip tones, but with hints of brightness and shine. Go easy on facial coloring and avoid heavily "rouged" looks. Creamy tones with just a slight flush of color are best.

For the going-gray brunette, nothing is more dramatic in fashion than white, black or combinations of both. Clear grays and some of the intense blues are eminently flattering. Not for brunettes is the pastel world; they may be the boldest of the going-grays. The radiant white-haired set should select colors to intensify and brighten eye color and play up the hair. Don't use shock colors that overpower the radiance of the hair; instead, choose clear, light colors—not the namby-pamby, almost no-color pastels and prints that are associated with age. Above all, the snowy head should be held with pride.

GRAY AND WHITE Q'S AND A'S

How can the purplish discoloration on my scalp and hair be avoided when I use a blue rinse to keep my hair silvery white?

Only old-fashioned "blueing" rinses produce staining of this nature and frequently rub off. Choose one of the modern rinses with names like "silver" or "white," which last from shampoo to shampoo and which are formulated especially for white and/or gray hair.

How can gray or white hair be treated to feel silkier and to look less strawlike?

Use a conditioner after shampooing. If the hair continues to feel coarse, a more intensive conditioning treatment with scalp massage before shampooing is necessary to improve texture and manageability.

Is it advisable to use a lightener on hair that is 50 percent white, so that the rest will match?

Never. A lightener alone would produce an unpleasant yellow on the pigmented hair. If left on long enough and in sufficient strength to remove all pigment, it would result in breakage of the hair shafts.

What causes yellow discoloration on white or light-gray hair?

Excessive heat—electric curlers, dryers set on high thermostat readings and too-hot water used during shampooing or rinsing—any one or all can be the cause. Perspiration from the scalp, especially during sleep, and improper use of permanent-wave solutions can also be the culprits.

How can the yellow be removed from the hair?

A deep conditioning treatment is the first step. Then a non-coating, non-staining silvery rinse designed for white hair should be applied.

What can be done about thin white hair through which the scalp shows? Would coloring it give it more body and make it feel thicker?

Coloring hair will give a better "hand" to the hair, making it feel thicker, but not to a great degree. A rinse to add highlights plus a short hairstyle with soft, open curls or waves will create an illusion of thicker hair.

Once hair has gone gray or white, is a consultation with a professional colorist necessary?

If the hair is gray—that is, half white and half natural pigmented color—consulting a professional colorist is a good idea. He or she can best advise whether to cover the gray or white hair to blend with the natural hair and whether to go to a lighter or darker shade. The colorist will also suggest where to add highlights and will advise you whether, for your lifestyle, you need permanent or merely temporary color. In the case of all white hair, the professional colorist can best recommend the kind of rinse, conditioning and maintenance your hair needs to promote shine and good texture and keep the hair an attractive white.

Why do the first gray hairs that appear seem to pop up from the rest of the hair and have a coarse, almost wiry texture? What can be done about them?

In the aging process, as hair loses its pigment and becomes white, its natural oil supply also begins to decrease. When that happens, the hair shafts become dry and lose their luster. The remedy is almost always deep conditioning treatments. The pop-up individual hairs may also need a very light misting of a fine, non-sticky hairdressing to keep them in place.

Is it true that if you pull out a gray hair when it appears, two will grow in its place?

No, that is definitely a myth.

Can hair turn white from shock or injury overnight?

This is another myth. There is no scientific evidence of this phenomenon. Injury to the roots of the hair, poor diet (especially one lacking in vitamin B), heredity and stress are the basic causes of white hair, which may appear in the very young as well as the old. Hair that is visible on the head and is naturally colored will retain that color until it is shed. It will not turn white. White hair, the result of the absence of melanin or pigment, is formed in the root or follicle of the hair and will be noticeable only after it has grown long enough to be seen.

What causes white hair to look brownish, often around the face?

Smoking can actually cause this, just as tar and nicotine can stain fingers. Also, pollutants in the atmosphere often have a bad effect on white and delicate blonde hair.

9

Special Effects

Highlights, streaks, shading in strategic strands, along with cal-
culated styling—these are the special artistries that can com-
pensate for nature's flaws and help to put your best face for-
ward.

The nuances of color in hair, as in fashion and makeup, can
be almost miraculous in correcting nature's errors by illusion.
Certain tricks of highlighting with selected strands and areas of
the hair are called "special effects." Carefully placed lighting
and shading—both in natural hair and in hair that has been
colored—can be most effective. Coupled with a well-designed
hairstyle, special effects can minimize faulty features and emphasize the best parts of the face and head. Together, for example, style and color, artfully employed, can camouflage such
less-than-perfect features as a nose that's too long, too large or
even too short; a face that's too full or too thin; a forehead too
low, too high or bulging; a chin that's too weak or too prominent, or a double chin; an uneven hairline; eyes too close together and too small. Unattractive face shapes can appear

closer to the ideal—the perfect oval—instead of being too round, too square, too long or too short. Whatever your individual problem, don't despair; look to your hair to correct your structural beauty faults in the easiest way.

Study the drawings and photographs in this chapter. See how a curl can conceal a feature, alter its appearance or divert the eye from it. Note the way a wave can hide, break a line, or deemphasize nature's imperfections. Observe the charm of a tendril that can lift, flatter and be the gayest deceiver of all. Study the way highlights around the face can give the illusion of width or height, or the way light-at-the-top draws the eye and makes a face appear slimmer, narrower or longer. Subtle lightening at the temples can make a too-high forehead seem lower or the eye area appear to be wider than it is.

Any way you look at it, the right hairstyle plus artful hair-color strategy offers a multitude of problem solvers. Add one more optical trick—makeup—and the mirror on your wall can surprise you with a wholly attractive vision you may never have dreamed possible. Problems you thought could only be resolved by costly and extensive cosmetic surgery are almost magically dissipated by illusion. The list below, together with the illustrations in this chapter, will help you zero in on the best way to solve your individual problem or problems. Then take action. First, get that all-important hairstyle, preferably by the most skilled stylist you can afford. Next, consult the very best colorist you can find. Even if you plan to do it yourself in the future, see a professional the first time around. Third, try the makeup techniques and tricks that further solve your problems. Fashion, of course, is the final fillip that turns the ugly duckling into a lovely swan. (Fashion notes and hints are to be found in the chapters on specific hair colors.)

Find, then, in the following, your particular beauty hang-up:

Long nose: It can be elegantly aristocratic, even beautiful in a classic Nefertiti way. Balance it, as Barbra Streisand does when she plays her most beautiful roles, with hair pulled back from the face and massed in a high or low chignon or an explosion of curls. Carry the eye up and away from the nose by having a special-effects lightening up from the brow. Never crowd the face with hair; this will only frame and emphasize the nose. Focus on eye makeup. Use a subtle dot of blusher on the tip of the nose to make it recede.

Large nose: Balance it with wide, curved waves, deftly highlighted to emphasize the sweep of them. Avoid tiny curls, short-short hairdos and fussy hair details. Use a darker foundation on the entire nose from that on the rest of the face to minimize it.

Short or too-tiny nose: This includes the "button" nose. It can be pert, saucy, even "cute," but with an overpowering mass of hair, the wearer can appear virtually "noseless." Opt for brief, caplike styles, with short curls, a feather cut, or a smooth gamine cut. Unless you are a dark brunette, keep your hair color on the light side, with special effects that shade the hair to lighter ends for pretty backlighting effects. Keep makeup light, simple and natural looking. Don't overemphasize eye or lip colors.

Too-wide nose: Keep hair coiffed to a just-below-eye-level length. Try the special effect of selected-strand lightening near the temples and up from the brow line. Place emphasis on eyes with makeup, and narrow the nose with the illusion of a stroke of dark contour-maker or blusher brushed on either side of it before applying overall makeup.

Too-full face: Highlight the hair at the top, up from the hairline across the brow, to draw attention there and help the face look slimmer, longer. Too-wide cheekbones, which make the face look fuller, can be made to look closer and the face slimmer with a coif that crowds and partially covers them. Try drawing deep, wide waves forward on the face to camouflage the widest and fullest parts. Create the illusion of a slim face with blusher or contour-maker, starting the color

71

high (mid-ear level), near the hairline, and drawing it on an angle to the center of the cheeks, then angling back again and down to mid-jawline. Feather and blend carefully.

Too-thin face: That "pinched" look can be dispelled with highlights placed at the sides, near the hairline, and shading outward so that the face seems wider at the cheekbone level. Wear a wide-winging style; keep hair length just below ear level. Large masses of hair will tend to make the face disappear. Thin-faced women have the advantage of giving the illusion that they are "all eyes." Make the most of this and emphasize eye makeup. Avoid severe styles, since thin faces tend to have a sharp look. Don't choose severely angled cuts. A curvy, rounded hairdo adds a softening effect.

Too-high forehead: Hair should be lighter at the temples, with highlights beginning a little way beyond the natural hairline at the top. Avoid slicked-back hairstyles and pony-tail

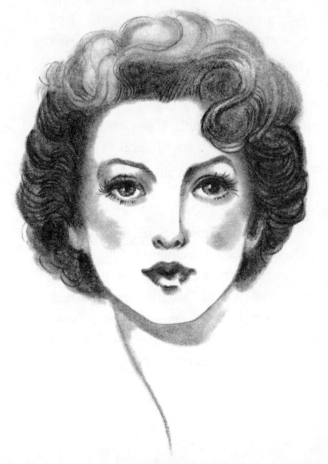

If your face is full, highlighting hair at the top is eye-lifting— and helps your face appear slimmer and longer.

effects. If you look well in them (and not everyone does) long, thick bangs or a bandeau of wave swooping low on the brow makes for the obvious cover-up. A *bulging brow* often is part of the one that's too high. The foregoing applies, *plus* the use of blusher or contour-maker lightly brushed across the bulging or most prominent areas before applying overall makeup.

The low brow: Add height with highlights, carefully placed all around the hairline from the front of the ears to the top of the brow. The strongest highlights are at the peak of the hairline, diminishing as they descend on either side of the face until they feather out to none at all. The hairstyle should crowd the face at eye-level and below, thereby lengthening the look of the brow. Lighter makeup toward the top will add height as well. If bangs are worn, they should be very, very brief and feathered up above the hairline for an inch or two. Small, tidy and close hairdos with an off-the-face line, plus the

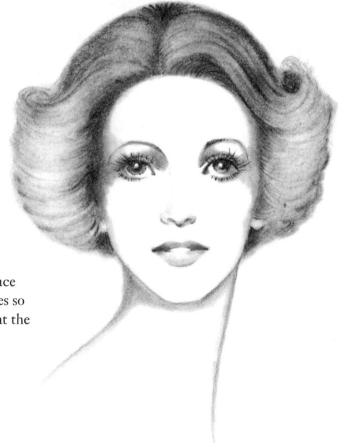

For a narrow face, place more highlights at sides so the face seems wider at the cheekbones.

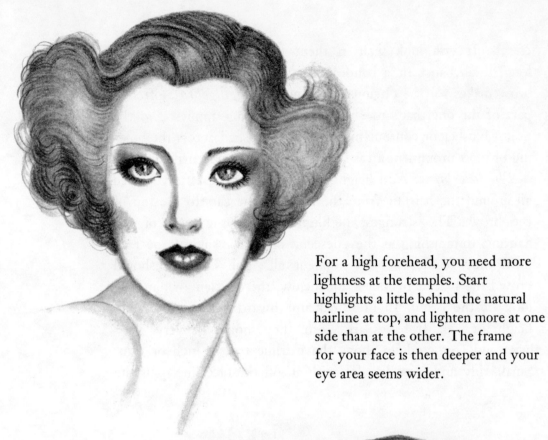

For a high forehead, you need more lightness at the temples. Start highlights a little behind the natural hairline at top, and lighten more at one side than at the other. The frame for your face is then deeper and your eye area seems wider.

When your forehead is low, put highlights at the front hairline for added height. This gives the illusion of a higher forehead.

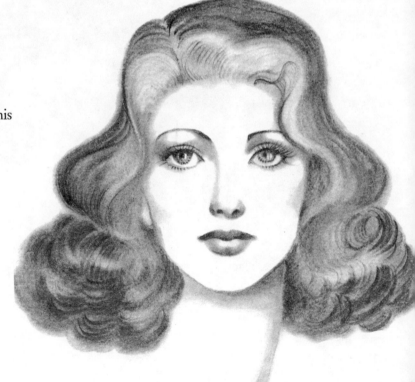

74

highlighting suggested, can hide the fact of the low forehead, too.

Problem chins: Weak ones can be strengthened by hairdos with fluffs of wave and curls below ear-level and drawn forward. Highlights, from eye-level to the top of the brow, should fan out from the hairline and lighter makeup should be applied to the chin for more prominence. *Jutting or too-pronounced* chins need the softening effect of medium-long hair, never pulled severely back, but crowding forward on the face. Highlighting moves toward the top to draw attention upward, and blusher or dark contour-maker should be worn on the chin under regular makeup. If short hair is desired, wear it brushed high and full on the top, full at the front. *Double chins* need both the look-up and chin-up treatment. Upswept coifs with highlighting to carry the eye aloft starts at the brow and sides and carries upward for added height and simple eye distraction. The wearer should try to keep the head and chin up to minimize the so-called "double chin."

Eyes too small, too close: Width-illusion is the essential here. Highlighting hair at the temples, hairstyles that are drawn back from the temples and fastened at the sides to swing loose, plus the use of illusory eye-makeup tricks (liners and shadows starting at the middle of the lids and extending beyond them; mascara applied more heavily to the outer edges of the lashes; brow ends extended) will create the look of larger, farther-apart eyes.

If none of the foregoing is your problem, count yourself fortunate indeed. On the other hand, perhaps your trouble is simply, or not so simply, your basic face shape. The perfect or ideal shape is oval, about in this proportion: five inches wide across the forehead, five and a half inches under the eyes, four and a half inches across just under the nose, three and a quarter inches wide under the mouth, and from chin tip to hairline at top of brow, seven and a half inches. These are flat, horizontal measurements. Use a ruler to find out how you measure up. If you're way off these proportions, you may find you're in one of the following problem categories: round, square, oblong or diamond.

The *round face* can appear more nearly oval when the hair is highlighted at the top, with selected strands lightened up from the hairline across the entire width of the brow. The illusory play of light will help to narrow the width of the roundness. The hair should be styled to crowd the face, thereby obscuring the width or roundness. Then use makeup as directed for the *too-full face*.

The *square face* also needs emphasis at the top to lengthen the overall look. Soften the square lines by adding height—with highlighting across the brow. Try curvy bangs if you can wear them, a diagonal part to offset the stark symmetry of squareness, or soft, full waves bracketing the brow. Soft fullness at the sides will also help. Never style hair with a severe, pulled-back-at-the-temples hairdo. Also, never have it too wide at the chin level. Avoid severe hairdos. Chances are that the jaw is too broad and blusher or contour-maker should be stroked lightly along and just under the jawline to help minimize it and soften the overall look.

The *oblong face*, long and narrow, squared at brow and chin, needs to have its length cut and softened. Consider a swoop of soft wave angled on the brow and a chin-length style that moves forward on the cheeks. Illusory highlighting at the temples feathered from the hairline back will create a wider look, hence shorten the length. Avoid sleek, pulled-back styles and coifs that add unwanted height. A low side part helps shorten the brow and round out corners if the brow is square. Use contour-maker at top of brow under makeup to diminish its height, and similarly on chin and jawline.

The *diamond face*, wide through the middle and narrow of brow with a pointy narrow chin, needs all the softness it can get to minimize the angular geometry. Lightened strands at the sides of the brow to help widen it, plus softness of style at the

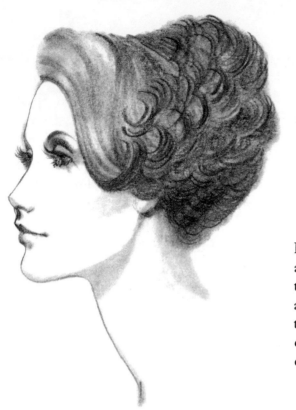

If you highlight your hair and want a permanent too, start curl behind the highlights, holding out the hair around your face. Front hair can then be used for a smooth look or can be rolled on curlers when all-over curl is wanted.

For subtle lighting in tinted hair, pull out random strands when you color it and then either lighten them separately or let them lighten naturally in sunlight.

sides to deemphasize the width of the cheekbones, begin the illusion of a rounded oval. A style just a bit below ear-length, curving up and forward on the cheeks, will narrow the span. If the head and all the features are diminutive and the chin is not too pointy, a very short, softly curled coif works nicely, with tendrils bracketing the brow. Lessen the angular effect of the diamond at the base by strengthening the jawline with a brush-on of whitener all around and blended with makeup foundation.

Remember that strategically placed streaks and shadings of the hair, with two and sometimes more colors, can help create symmetry for a face that's not ideally proportioned. The effect should always be soft and natural—never streaky and harsh, never obvious. Most of the special effects achieved through highlighting are done around or near the face, where hair, by nature, is usually lighter. The subtle extension of these normal plays of light, taking advantage of nature's way to create illusions, is what special effects are all about. Hair does not grow all in a single color; it is many colors, as we have seen. It is up to you and your colorist to bring forth its best hues, playing up the lights that give new dimensions of beauty for the most attractive look possible.

10

Some Special Problems

Blaming hair damage on coloring is a gross error. That and other special problems go deeper than the tints, toners and lighteners so carefully formulated to make your hair healthier and more beautiful.

The individual who regularly patronizes an expert coloring salon probably has the healthiest scalp and hair in the world. Rarely does she or he have dandruff and other scalp disorders, excessive falling hair, split ends, too-dry hair or too-oily hair. However, that is true only if a program of sound maintenance is practiced between colorings and stylings. Problems arise for other reasons—not as a result of the coloring process itself; they are most often due to poor health, poor judgment or lack of the proper information.

In the following collection of most-often-asked questions, find your individual problem or problems, how to understand and solve them, and how to avoid them in the future:

Does anesthesia used during surgery change the color of tinted hair?

No. The anesthesia would have to leak into the atmosphere in order to affect coloring. What may affect the color, especially near the roots of the hair, is excessive perspiration on the scalp during the stress of surgery. The acidity in perspiration could darken lightened hair or produce red tones.

Does permanent waving or hair straightening affect hair coloring?

When one has had any chemical treatment, such as straightening or relaxing the hair or permanent waving, it is best to have at least one or two shampoos and conditioning treatments before attempting coloring. Chemically treated hair is highly absorbent and after, say, a fresh permanent, the coloring agent should be diluted with water, worked through the hair and left on for less time than normal. Otherwise the color will penetrate too quickly and will look too heavy and deep, especially on hair ends. Using water to dilute the color is a must; do *not* use shampoo for the purpose.

Will a hair dryer affect hair coloring?

It is best never to use a very hot dryer on any hair, tinted or natural. Never use a hot dryer immediately after coloring, because the color will sometimes fade before it has had a chance to set. If one is home and there is time, best results are achieved when the hair dries naturally. Otherwise, towel-dry, without rubbing too vigorously, before setting, combing or otherwise styling.

Just how safe is hair coloring?

Perfectly safe. A few years ago some inconclusive research indicated that hair tints might have harmful chemicals in them. Even though there is no proof of this, the major manufacturers of hair-coloring products have voluntarily reformulated all of their products to eliminate even potentially controversial ingredients. Every user of these or any other beauty and health products should always follow use directions to the letter to ensure successful results.

Is it a fact that hair coloring won't take during pregnancy and that it should be postponed until afterward?

Not at all. That's like saying permanent waves aren't successful when administered during pregnancy. Coloring, with its accompanying conditioners to maintain the health of the hair, can, in fact, be very beneficial to the hair during pregnancy. Hair coloring can provide a psychological boost, too, since this is a time when a woman needs to look and feel her loveliest and healthiest.

Why is there sometimes excessive hair loss after pregnancy?

This is really an illusion. Hair is constantly growing and shedding, more at certain seasons of the year and at certain stages of life. During pregnancy, hormonal balances shift and hair often grows more thickly and rapidly. Afterward, as the body returns to normal, the extra hair growth is shed and normal growth patterns are reestablished.

Sometimes when I apply lightener to my hair my scalp burns, tingles and itches. Why does this happen?

You may be combing or brushing your hair too vigorously on the day the lightener is applied, thereby irritating your scalp. You may be shampooing your hair just before lightening it, or using a hot blow-dryer. Too much tension on the hair—as in blow-drying and styling—can make the scalp sensitive. Perhaps your shampoo is too strong. Sometimes when the scalp is very dry, just adding a shampoo will cause painful burning and itching. You may be using a too-harsh, old-fashioned lightener. Any of these can cause a reaction. The problem may be very simply solved by switching to a gentler shampoo or a more modern, creamy lightener. There is also the possibility that you may be developing a sensitivity to the product. A patch test should be made and, if sensitivity is indicated, lightening should be discontinued for a while.

Do birth control pills affect the color of the hair?

No, but in some cases women will experience a slight loss of hair while taking the pills.

Is it all right to have hair tinted during the menstrual period, and will the coloring take properly?

The coloring will definitely take properly, but since some women develop a skin sensitivity at this time—not an allergic reaction, but a reddening of the skin—it may be best to postpone coloring until a day or two afterward or a day or two before, if you are prone to that kind of sensitivity.

What about medications? Can they affect coloring results?

No, but certain medications can change an individual's skin sensitivity, similarly to what sometimes occurs during the menstrual period.

Why does tinted hair often change to an unattractive color when it has been exposed to swimming-pool water?

It doesn't always, but the chemical levels in some swimming pools are so high that delicately tinted hair can suffer unwanted changes. It is important that the hair always be cleansed after a swim—not necessarily with a shampoo, but simply by flushing it with lots of clear, fresh water to carry off pool- and/or salt-water residue and chemical deposits.

If one is allergic to most hair colorings, what should be used? How about vegetable dyes?

Vegetable dyes were the earliest ever used, thousands of years ago; the results were unnatural and streaky, or very matte. Today, henna is the only vegetable color available, but it, too, produces an unnatural red shade, dully coating the hair and giving a harsh effect. Try a temporary color rinse that is non-allergenic instead.

Can a human-hair wig or hairpiece be successfully lightened or tinted at home?

Not usually, since this is extremely difficult to do while keeping the foundation from becoming saturated and the hair strands from being loosened. Human-hair wigs and hairpieces can be lightened, tinted and, of course, cleansed. It is best to have a professional do the coloring for these fairly expensive accessories, though.

I wear glasses in order to see what I'm doing when I color my hair, but the sidepieces always leave horizontal streaks where the coloring can't reach. How can I remedy this?

Correct the streaks by brushing a diluted tint mixture on after the rest of the hair has been treated and you have removed your glasses for the last minute.

Can hair be colored so that it precisely matches any color on the manufacturer's chart?

Only an artist at hair coloring could duplicate those shades exactly on an individual's hair. Home hair colorists can only approximate. The colors on the chart were made from photographs of hair that was pure white before being tinted, so unless one plans to remove all natural color from the hair first, it is best to choose one shade lighter than that desired. Remember, too, that the chart colors are opaque, with no light shining through as in the actual hair. Therefore, the chart colors will be a shade or two darker than in real life.

Can lighteners formulated for the hair on one's head also be used to lighten dark facial hair?

It is never advisable to use lighteners for the hair on the head to lighten facial hair. There are special products designed for facial hair bleaching; these should be used according to the manufacturer's instructions. Do a small patch test first before applying the product to larger areas.

What about using hair-coloring products on brows and lashes?

In more and more states, the use of hair tints on brows and lashes is against the law. Users of hair-coloring products are cautioned in the use directions to keep the products away from the eyes. Therefore, it is wiser to use cosmetics to achieve the effects desired for brows and lashes.

What causes hair colorings to fade and grow dull with repeated shampoos? Can one shampoo the hair too often?

Check the shampoo you are using. It should be specifically formulated for tinted or lightened hair and the label should specify that it does not strip color. This should be a gentle, creamy, non-detergent type (detergent shampoos strip oil from the hair and lift off some of the color). Be sure to follow with a good conditioner, also formulated to guard the delicate tones of hair colors. Hair will be brightest, liveliest and most easy to manage when it is clean and conditioned. No, you cannot wash your hair too often.

Will heat curlers hurt hair coloring?

Too much heat of any kind is not kind to the hair, whether it's natural or tinted. When it is necessary to use heat rollers, put a little protective conditioner on the ends of the hair and use end papers before winding each one. Extremely hot rollers not only will dry out porous hair ends, but will fade and change the more subtle and delicate colors to a markedly noticeable degree.

What are the best kinds of rollers?

Those that are very smoothly finished produce the smoothest styles without tangling or breaking the hair. Use setting lotions sparingly, for special occasions and special fullness of style. Beware of hair sprays. For hard-to-hold hair, sparing use—just a light misting—of a gentle spray with color-guarding properties is permissible.

What can be done to prevent staining of the skin when using dark tints?

Protect the skin with a light protective cream or petroleum jelly. Apply it around the hairline, cover the backs of the ears and, if you're a spatterer, apply it to the entire face and neck area. If the scalp has any small cuts or abrasions, coat this area, too, before applying color.

11

What Color for Teens?

Part of being very young is being versatile—eager to experiment, explore and change. Go easy on the color; vary the hairdo instead.

During childhood, the most popular dolls are blonde; hence little girls identify with light hair and they, as well as many of their mothers, often yearn for what we call the Barbie-doll look. Most Caucasian children are born blonde or blondish, ranging from nearly white-blonde or "towheaded" to a reddish gold or a light brown flecked with gold. How long that hair stays in the blonde category depends on the child's heredity factors as well as on the thickness and texture of the hair. For the most part, the true blonde has fine, wispy, silken hair. The longest-lasting blonde is the golden, almost reddish blonde, because that type keeps its highlights and brightness longer. It is also, in general, heavier in texture than the short-lasting towhead type. The latter, the nearly white-blonde, is almost totally devoid of pigment and tends to fade into a nondescript brown quicker than any other color—what is sometimes called a "dirty blonde," characterized by a flat, dull appearance.

Too many eager mothers ambitiously try to keep their little golden-haired girls blonde; the soft, shining hair of childhood is too soon subjected to home-coloring efforts, which can often be abusive to young (or any other) hair. Until the middle to late teens, a child's hair, in almost every case, should be left natural. Its only care should be that of a scrupulous cleansing regimen with periodic trimming and shaping to maintain health and beauty. Only in the rare cases of totally unattractive, dull and flat hair color should nature be tampered with. In those instances, the rule is: Hold off as long as possible, yielding only when the hair is so unattractive as to be a psychological problem for the young girl. At that point a professional should be consulted. Home-brewed rinses and remedies are not advisable. The better way, of course, is to encourage plenty of outdoor exercise in the sunshine. The sun easily lightens and brightens young hair with a specially wonderful glow and shine.

A young girl's desire to experiment not only with her hairstyle but with hair coloring is natural, but until the mid-teens she will be wisest to confine herself to *styling*. In that department she has a wide world of choice—switching parts, fashioning braids and pony tails, looping, overlapping, gently curling here and there, and accessorizing her locks with combs, bows, flowers or pretty barrettes. Experiments with home haircutting are not advisable. Most young girls prefer long hair—especially those who have straight or wavy hair. On the young, long hair can be most attractive, provided it is professionally trimmed regularly (just the ends, in most cases) and maintained with scrupulous cleanliness. Short and very short hairstyles are beguiling on the young, and are especially appropriate for the girl with very curly hair. In this case, a professional cut and shaping is a must. Above all, the adolescent should never have bangs and should try to adopt hairstyles that keep the hair off the brow and face, if at all possible. These are the so-called "acne years," when hair covering the facial skin encourages and aggravates the condition, particularly in cases where the scalp is excessively oily.

When the hair is mousy and drab and coloring is the only answer, see a good colorist. The first step for young hair should be simply a lightening and softening of the hair with the resultant look of sunstruck locks. The easiest way is having subtle shadings of highlights with the lighter color framing the face. This lessens the possibility of regrowth showing too quickly and should not need to be redone more than two or three times a year, as the seasons change—perhaps not at all during the summer, if the hair is exposed daily to strong sunlight. The sun, when hair is in good condition, will enhance the color, lightly fading it but not removing it altogether. If, however, the hair is in poor condition, abused with bleaching, overpermanenting or relaxing, or if it is very delicate and fragile, excessive exposure to strong sun will intensify the damage, which can only be undone with an intensive reconditioning program.

If the impulse to try home hair coloring is irresistible, the best course is first to try a temporary rinse, one that lasts only from shampoo to shampoo and readily washes out. The color will not penetrate the hair shaft and will have less clarity than permanent coloring, but it will satisfy the urge to change and can produce some pretty effects if intelligently used. Before making a selection, study the natural hair. Look at a strand held up before the light, preferably with a magnifying glass. There will be many different colors, since hair is never all one shade. Is it predominantly gold, red-gold, warm brown, or what? Snip a few inconspicuous strands from the back of the head, a few more from the side near the face (long strands, not ends, which may be dried out, split and faded). There will be a distinct difference; hair is usually darkest at the nape of the neck or at the lower back of the head, and lighter around the face. Spread the strands on a piece of white paper under strong light and look at these through a magnifying glass. Now decide which shades dominate and which would be most desirable. Then consult the color chart of the temporary rinse. Choose a color that's most like the hair samples in the preferred strands. Next, carefully read the instructions and, again, experiment before making the plunge. Choose a few strands near the face. Apply the color, following directions to the letter, then let the strand dry completely. (This will take only a few minutes if the hair is towel-blotted and dried.) If all is satisfactory, proceed with the whole head.

Next step on the ladder of coloring for the older teen could be a semipermanent color, actually a light staining type of rinse that can enrich and highlight the hair. Choose a color almost identical to the natural hair (studying the hair as noted, with strong light and a magnifying glass), but with either a golden light to it or a little bit of reddish highlight. Follow the directions meticulously, first doing an experimental strand to see if it is the color desired before doing the rest of the hair. This coloring will give a lustrous shine as well as bringing out a warm highlight. The natural color will not be greatly changed, so there will be no ugly regrowth period. If this type of coloring is discontinued, the hair won't look neglected as it grows out. The conditioning quality of these colors can help bring hair back to beauty when it has been damaged with bleach; the color will tone down the harsh orangey cast and help restore silkiness as the hair grows back to its natural color.

Remember, young hair is almost always beautiful hair. The worst thing a teen can do is to start bleaching her hair at fourteen or fifteen years of age. Harsh streaks and tipping at any age look artificial and ugly; on a thirteen-year-old, frankly, they look ridiculous. Healthy young hair is the most beautiful of all, envied by older women. It should be guarded as one of the most priceless assets of youth and treated with the same care as a young skin and a young body.

What does painting the hair mean?

Hair painting is a technique that involves taking very small strands of hair, lightening them a few shades as the sun would and giving a very gentle highlighted, sunny look. The effect is natural and especially becoming if the hair is blonde and just becoming a so-called "dirty blonde." It is also extremely effective on light-brown hair that is tending toward an all-over flat-looking brown. It should be done extremely carefully—less instead of more—and only on a seasonal basis, when the hair is not being exposed to the sun and is beginning to look dull and flat in some areas while still appearing shiny and lustrous in others.

Can it be done at home?

Yes, but extremely carefully, taking very small strands of hair (anywhere from three to six hairs) and using only a little bit of the color-lightening product. The substance used is very thick and pasty and will stay right where it's applied, without perceptibly affecting the rest of the hair. In a sense, it's a lot like finger painting; you can do it with your fingers in some cases, or with a brush. The substance has an almost gel-like consistency; using the fingers works best, because you can pick out narrower strands for a better effect. The lightener is very gentle, doesn't add color and should be applied so that it doesn't touch the roots of the hair at all. That way there will be no perceptible new growth in the ensuing weeks.

Will lemon juice lighten the hair? Is it harmful?

Yes, lemon juice can lighten the hair a little bit, but it dries out the hair and tends to strip the natural oil coating from it. In the very young, this will take away natural shine and leave a dull finish. During adolescence, when hair and skin tend to be oily, even greasy, both vinegar with its acidity and lemon juice in the last rinse water will remove the excess oiliness. There are, however, so many excellent products on the market today that are so much more beneficial that one doesn't need to resort to home remedies.

Is camomile tea a suitable lightener?

Camomile is an old-fashioned rinse and, like other such vegetable products, it acts as a stain of a very mild nature, adding little or nothing to the hair.

Just how bad is peroxide for the hair?

Peroxide is one of the agents used in lightening hair and should be applied by a skilled technician. One of the most common mistakes that young girls make is using peroxide alone as a lightener and letting it dry in the hair. Done to any extent and repeatedly, this not only will dry out the hair to the point of disintegration, it will bring out ugly yellow and orange casts. Peroxide, used professionally, is combined with other agents that protect the hair during the lightening process. This is the case, too, with well-formulated consumer products for home hair lightening.

What about laundry bleach to keep blonde hair blonde?

Some of these are so strong that the naked eye can see the hair disintegrate. Nothing could be more harmful to the hair and scalp, young or old. Aside from producing hair that is so dry it crackles, color that daily grows more unattractive in its orangey brassiness and totally lifeless hair, using laundry bleach can be dangerous—to the scalp, and to the eyes if it gets near them. Think of putting a piece of fine fabric in full-strength laundry bleach and letting it dry; the fibers in the fabric will be weakened and eaten away. Think, then, of your hair as your fine fabric accessory—and be gentle with it.

Would it be all right to use her mother's hair lightener on a six- or seven-year-old girl whose blonde hair is turning darker?

91

Lightening children's hair with grown-ups' products is never recommended. Not only might these products, though safe for adult hair, damage fine young hair, but they may also injure tender young scalps. When the young blonde-turning-brunette girl is old enough—usually in the upper teen range—to decide what color she prefers, she may choose one of the gentler methods of lightening. Meanwhile, keep the child's hair clean —freshly shampooed hair always appears lighter—and gently brushed to encourage shine, and let her enjoy experimenting with hairdo changes now and then.

Can hair be washed too much?

Never. Probably one of the healthiest things young girls do for their hair—and their skin—is to shampoo it every day or so. Often the teen has a skin problem, which can be accentuated by oil in the hair rubbing off on the face, especially during sleep. Of course, a very gentle shampoo must be used on young hair, and during the teen years a mild conditioner is a must. It imparts shine and manageability and offsets the effects of hair dryers, heat curlers and other appliances used for grooming or styling.

Is it necessary to brush a child's hair a full hundred strokes?

No. As a matter of fact, too much and the wrong kind of brushing (that is, too vigorously and with nylon-bristle brushes) can be harmful, pulling too much on the baby-fine hair shafts. Both for adults and the young, a little brushing goes a long way. It is better to massage the scalp with the fingertips to loosen the skin, promote circulation and help distribute the oil along the hair shaft. Follow up with a light brushing to further disperse the oil and thereby encourage shine.

What is the best way to shampoo young hair?

Use a gentle shampoo, followed by a tepid, nearly cool rinsing with clear water. Then the hair should be towel-dried, with a massaging kind of use of the towel. Comb through the hair with a wide-toothed comb, never with a brush. Dry it naturally, if possible, in the air, or with slight help from an electric blower—set on cool or warm, never hot. Do not go to bed with wet hair, and never with rollers in your hair. Wet hair is much more fragile than dry, and the pressure from sleeping will leave unsightly marks in a setting.

What about braiding hair, especially in skinny braids?

Hair should be completely dry when braided and should not be worn in braids every day. Just as a tight pony tail worn daily will cause breakage from traction, so, too, can braids. Young hair is pretty when it's long and swinging; the constant circulation of air and light through the hair makes it even more attractive. Now and then a special style for a special event can be fun—e.g., the Botticelli look, which needs a very young face to carry it off. Try it once in a long while only; it is not for everyday wear. While the hair is slightly damp, make tiny braids all over the head. When the hair is thoroughly dry, gently brush it out for a very full look.

How long should a young girl wear her hair? When is it too long?

Just below shoulder-length is the most beautiful. Too-long hair tangles easily and gets in the way during sports, dancing, etc. When hair is left alone to grow as long as possible, the ends will be "old" hair, which is usually dry and prone to split or frizz. Trimmed regularly, long hair will have more bounce and will look healthier and shinier.

What if the hair is too curly, frizzy, almost kinky?

This, when the fashion for long, smooth or wavy hair is so popular, can be very distressing for a young girl. For the most part, curly hair is prettier when worn very short in a halo of soft curls. On the rarest occasions, when a young girl's hair is so tightly kinky as to be unmanageable and it has become a strong psychological problem for the girl, then a professional consultation on relaxing the hair is recommended. Setting the damp hair on very large rollers which almost stretch the hair will work between shampoos on some over-curly hair—or turban-wrap it with a scarf while it is damp and combed smooth. When thoroughly dry, it will comb out relatively smoothly.

Only when all methods that don't apply heat (hot combs, pressing, et al.) or chemicals have been exhausted should hair-straightening—or hair relaxing, as it is often called—be explored. Young hair, especially the truly kinky variety, is fine and fragile, much more susceptible than any other to harsh treatment. Put this off as long as possible until the girl is older. Then be sure that the relaxer, straightener or permanent-in-reverse (most chemicals used are those formulated for permanent waving) is the gentlest and mildest available to begin with. Follow directions to the letter, if this is not being professionally done, and be sure to make a strand test first to ensure against hair damage.

What causes frizzy hair on normally manageable young hair? How can it be corrected?

Excessive dryness due to harsh shampoos, any lightening or permanenting agents used repeatedly, climate, pool water or salt water that is not rinsed out immediately after exposure, poor health, tension, poor diet—any or all of these can cause frizziness. If the condition is very bad, then deep conditioning treatments, at least once a week, are recommended. A mild case of frizzy, unruly, unmanageable hair, of course, should be treated with frequent use of a gentle shampoo and a conditioner.

Will hair sprays help?

Not really, and a teen should hardly ever have any reason to use hair spray. A few wispy, flying ends on soft young hair can be very pretty; sprays would only stiffen and coat them.

Aside from trimming them off, what else can be done about split ends?

Conditioning on a regular basis will smooth them together—not eliminate them—so that they do not appear to be split.

What if a young girl has a faulty hairline—a too-low or a too-high one? Could hair coloring work to correct this by illusion as it does in adults?

It is definitely not advisable. Until a girl is old enough—somewhere around seventeen or eighteen—hairstyling to camouflage faulty hairlines should be the only solution to the problem.

BASIC TEEN TABOOS

Braids and pony tails on a constant basis.
Pressing or ironing the hair.
Wearing a part constantly in the same place.
Heat rollers for setting too often.
Using setting lotions and hair sprays too much.
Amateur bleaches and coloring: peroxide, ammonia, laundry bleach, lemon juice, vinegar, carbon paper.
Any all-over color that will change the natural coloring drastically. Anything that colors the root area.
Metallic and wire rollers; any that are not smooth.
Complicated adult hairdos.

Remember, less is the most for teen-age hair.

12

Color Him, Too

Men, too, are turning back the calendar with more sophisticated grooming aids—and one of the most important is discreet, subtle hair coloring.

In nature, except among humans, the male of the species is invariably more colorful than the female. Predominantly, it has been the women who utilized the arts of adornment while the man addressed himself to business and war. Occasionally, in the course of history, men have tried to outdo women with elaborate wigs and plumage, but for the most part they have been the drabber of the species in the matter of dress and embellishment. Today, though men remain more understated in their garb and subtler in their grooming, they are not without color —in their clothing and, yes, in their hair.

More and more men are borrowing the sensible skin- and hair-care aids that women have used for decades—the good shampoos and hair conditioners, the face- and body-cleansing agents, the skin revitalizers and toners. Even fresh, masculine scents are an essential part of the twentieth-century man's grooming wardrobe. It is all part of a deeply rooted desire to remain youthful and healthy as long as possible.

Those universally dreaded signs of aging—graying and the loss of hair—have led ever-larger numbers of men to explore hair coloring, hair transplants and hairpieces. They have enjoyed ever-increasing success as the providers of these services have become more expert than ever before. Today the well-turned-out man has a hair stylist, not just the corner barber who crops and chops, ignoring the face below. It is no longer uncommon for a man to consult his stylist about "touching up" those first signs of gray or having a "highlight" rinse for hair that's beginning to go drab and lackluster. Complete color changes are not uncommon, and more than one major company in this country underwrites the cost of coloring, transplants and hairpieces so that its salesmen will look their best. The astute executive knows that while the race often is to the young and the swift in business, it is on the mature, experienced employee that he most often relies. Public figures—politicians, actors, commentators and performers by the hundreds —know the merits of hair coloring for men. Can one imagine a balding Frank Sinatra, for instance, or a thin-on-top Johnny Carson? It is not vanity or false pride for a man to tint his hair or to wear an undetectable hairpiece. The well-groomed, youthful-looking man gains not only in the impression he makes on others, but in his own self-esteem—and that extra dimension of attractiveness actually is easily acquired.

Whether a man is a beginner or an old hand at coloring, a temporary-rinser or a permanent-color user, he must be even more careful than a woman when choosing and using color. *All* types of men's hair coloring should be very subtle and soft. Anything that looks harshly bright or artificial in any way should be avoided. The very first step should be to make the hair look a little lighter and a bit brighter, a little sunnier, with a little more shine added to it. If beginning gray is the problem, then a color close to the original hair color should be used. Usually the best results are achieved with a semipermanent coloring that does not contain peroxide, and that is two or three shades lighter than the natural color. If the hair is a dark brown, a lighter, softer brown will be most effective. The grays should be blended in, but not every single gray hair should be covered, since a few of these will add to the highlights and to the illusion of shine. If the hair is very gray, leaving the little temple hairs uncolored will look more natural and, as the hair grows out, a regrowth line will be unnoticeable. Sideburns should be kept a little darker as a frame and shaping for the face, but they should not be too long, since regrowth shows very quickly in this area.

Styling is extremely important when hair is colored; a slightly fuller, longer style is best so that new growth is not too obvious. Getting a cut and shaping on a regular basis, rather than letting the hair get shaggy and then having it trimmed, will always keep hair in better condition and show off color most attractively. Generally, hair looks better in wintertime if it is a bit fuller, because bulkier clothes are worn then.

Hair, colored or natural, should always be kept very clean. No man or woman goes bald from excessive showering or shampooing. Use of the appropriate shampoo for the type of hair (normal, dry, oily, colored) is important, however. Shampooing daily does not hurt, but the shampoo must always be followed with a conditioner. Always shampoo after swimming (especially in chlorinated water) and after tennis, jogging or any form of exercise. Hair should be towel-dried thoroughly before you begin to blow it dry. Then use some kind of protective conditioner—a light, moisturizing lotion—while the hair is being blown dry, so that it doesn't get burned by the blower, thus losing its sheen and luster.

Radical changes in hair color—say, from sandy to dark brunette or from brown to red—are not advisable for men. Women, in many instances, can have more-or-less extreme changes because they have more of a mass of hair and because they can complement the new coloring with makeup. A man does not wear makeup; his only accessory is his hair. If it's a non-color—a gray or white—it can often wash out his whole appearance. Very often a man will prematurely go gray while women of comparable age do not—yet a woman can be dazzling, thanks to makeup and fashion, with prematurely gray hair. For most men, gray hair simply adds years to their ages. Since men's hair coloring has become quite accepted now, why shouldn't a man opt for the most youthful appearance he can achieve, for as long as he can.

MEN'S COLORING Q's AND A's

Why does new growth show so much more quickly on a man's hair than on a woman's when the hair has been colored?

Usually a man's hair is kept much shorter and shaped much closer to the head. Also, most men wear some kind of part, while a woman has a choice of many partless hairstyles to conceal the lines of regrowth.

Does a man's hair grow faster than a woman's and will it therefore need more frequent recoloring?

Not necessarily. A rule of thumb is that the average person's hair—male or female—grows at the rate of half an inch per month. The more active and the healthier an individual is, the more rapidly the hair grows. There are also times of the year when hair grows faster—summer, for instance, when people are out of doors and engaged in more physical activity. It all has to do with health.

What about excessive shedding and resultant thinning or balding of the hair? Are men prone to this more than women?

Shedding is a normal process, the average being about eighty to one hundred hair strands per day. It, too, is a seasonal occurrence and frequently is dictated by one's physical condition.

Diet deficiencies can cause excessive fall-out; so, too, can lack of exercise, fatigue, stress and tension of all kinds. Men and women are equally prone to excessive shedding when bad health is the culprit. Checking with a physician in this case is the answer; only a doctor can determine vitamin deficiencies or diet problems and prescribe accordingly.

Would a man who has thin, fine hair benefit by having a permanent?

Yes, but it is best done by a professional; men, unlike women, seem not to have the knack or the patience for home-administered permanents or hair straightening. The permanent should be one designed for body; it can do wonders when expertly handled. (If it is overdone, the hair frizzes.)

Will hair coloring make thin hair look thicker?

Again, in the hands of an expert, hair coloring can fool the eye, making hair seem denser and in many cases actually adding body to thin hair. Going lighter in coloring, rather than darker, will lessen the visible contrast between the strands of hair and the scalp. A good cut with layered shaping will also give the illusion of more, thicker hair.

What about too-curly hair?

A smoother shape to the hair can be achieved with a relaxer —a permanent, in other words, designed to straighten the hair —but go easy. Again, let an expert do this. And, if hair coloring is to be done, wait a few weeks after having the hair relaxed before having it lightened or tinted.

If hair is going unbecomingly gray, what is the best color to choose in covering it?

If the hair originally was a nondescript, in-between shade— for example, a mousy brown, which is the average color for most men—a dark, sandy blonde—almost a light brown—with an ash tone would be a good choice. It should be very subtle.

How should salt-and-pepper gray hair be treated?

This kind of gray hair can be very attractive, both on younger and older men. The light part—the so-called gray, which is actually white hair that appears to be gray—must be kept very shiny, almost like platinum. There are numerous types of gray toners for men as well as women (either will work equally well on a man's hair) that will keep the gray parts sparkly white and will also keep those gray strands from popping up in a coarse, dry way. Whether the hair is streaked with gray, salt-and-pepper or all gray, it should be kept meticulously clean at all times and conditioned regularly after shampooing to keep it shining.

What kind of toner should be used?

Only the very light, almost whitening, kind of gray rinse with no blue cast whatsoever. A bluish tint is too obvious on a man's short hair and immediately creates an artificial effect.

Is that a temporary rinse?

Semipermanent kinds of coloring in the very-light-gray category, which are formulated for women but can readily be used by men, work best. Colorings that are sulfur- or metallic-based are not generally acceptable for men, because they leave a flat coating that dulls the hair. If a man tends to have scalp perspiration when he exercises, those colorings create an offensive sulfur-like odor in the hair.

Does hair coloring promote dandruff?

Quite the contrary. People who have their hair tinted and who care for it in the approved way—with proper shampooing and conditioning—usually have very clean, healthy scalps, which are not dry and flaky. True dandruff—not merely the shedding and flaking of a super-dry scalp—is a disease and is best treated by a dermatologist.

Will lightening the hair cause breakage and split ends?

Not if it is done properly, with professional care. Breakage and split ends indicate that the hair shafts have been damaged, either by excessive exposure to heat (sun, hair dryers, hair blowers), overprocessing (straightening or permanent-waving improperly) or excessive bleaching—that is, the wrong kinds and techniques of hair coloring.

Will coloring the hair hasten baldness?

No. Hair loss is more prevalent among men and more noticeable because of the length of the hair. Balding is mostly hereditary, but one can retard it by keeping the scalp healthy, loose and flexible. Massage it with the fingertips to promote circulation, and don't let it get dry and flaky. Exercise is very important and, again, so is diet, with the B vitamins particularly important to hair growth. Be especially careful with weight-loss diets; check with a physician to be sure that a slimming diet is not omitting essential nutrients and vitamins.

When should one become disturbed about hair loss? How much is too much in the comb?

Extreme hair loss does not mean a few strands of hair in the comb. Nor does it mean the half-dozen hairs that come out when hair is wet and during shampooing. However, when a hand run over the top of the dry head with just a little stroking leaves a number of hairs in the hand and this continues for more than three or four weeks, it is time to see a physician for a complete physical checkup. If no physical problems are discovered, a dermatologist should be consulted.

Can medication produce hair loss?

Certain kinds of medication, as well as chemotherapy, can cause hair loss. When medication is discontinued, normal hair growth usually returns.

DO'S AND DON'TS

Do set a styling comb or blower on warm or cool when shaping the hair after it has been colored, especially on delicately toned and gray hair. Excessive heat and exposure to too-intense sun can alter the new color, making it brassy or faded.

DON'T have hair colored very, very dark, almost black. It not only will look artificial on most heads and with most complexions, but the very dark colors are difficult to maintain, taking on an unattractive reddish cast very rapidly.

Do protect gray or white hair from yellowing. Use only rinses that don't produce a coating on the hair. Wear a hat in tropical climates or when exercising outdoors in intense sunlight. Always shampoo, or at least rinse, hair thoroughly in clear water after swimming in salt or chlorinated water. Avoid colognes and hair preparations with fragrance; these can discolor or yellow the hair.

Do use a conditioner after shampooing gray or white hair, to prevent its becoming wiry and coarse-feeling.

DON'T go all out for a color change without being sure that your choice is both appropriate and attractive. When uncertain, try a wash-in, wash-out temporary rinse to determine the effect before going into a more permanent coloring.

Do consult a professional for best results, especially if toning and shading of selected hair strands is desired. A professional colorist can also create a natural pattern of shadings in the hair to compensate for facial irregularities, just as hair coloring is used to correct face shapes on women—for example, lightening certain areas to offset a too-low forehead, a too-wide or too-low brow, etc.

Do have a patch test before a first-time hair coloring. Men, as well as women, sometimes are allergic to certain hair-coloring products.

13

A Hair-Coloring Glossary

It's a wise head that knows basic hair-coloring terms. If you are exploring the possibility of a change of color, having your first consultation with a colorist or embarking on a do-it-yourself coloring, study these terms for a better understanding of the processes involved:

Allergy test: Also known as a *patch test* or *skin test.* Important for first-time coloring, this test is administered prior to coloring to determine possible allergic or hypersensitive reaction to certain coloring substances. It is made on a small patch of clear skin, usually on an inner arm or on the back of the neck.

Ash: A pale or "cool" shade as in "ash blonde" or "ash brown." Directly opposed to "warm" or bright tones.

Bleach: An old-fashioned word meaning to lighten the hair by removing pigmentation; also an agent for lightening.

Blend: A combination of ingredients or preparations; a mixture of integrated ingredients. Also, *blending,* the process of evening color throughout a strand of hair.

Brassy: Excess red, orange or brass color, giving a harsh, unnatural look. This most often occurs on blonde or red hair that has been inexpertly colored or that has been exposed to excessive heat.

Coating: The deposit on the outer surface of the hair (as opposed to penetrating color) by such methods of coloring as spraying, crayoning or temporary rinsing. Excessive amounts produce a lusterless, matte effect on the hair.

Color shampoo: Also sometimes called a *shampoo tint.* Applied like a shampoo, it contains cleansing agents as well as ingredients to highlight and subtly tint or enrich the natural hair color.

Color test: The treatment of a strand of hair with a proposed color formula prior to treating the entire head. Used to determine suitability of a formula and to check timing.

Colorfast shampoo: A mild shampoo specially formulated to cleanse and protect color-treated hair.

Colorist: A professional hairdresser who specializes in the application, care and maintenance of hair color. A highly skilled colorist is also an expert in special color effects.

Concentrate: Any hair preparation—shampoo, coloring agents, tints, etc.—designed to be diluted (usually with water) before use.

Condition: Often done before and/or during coloring, as well as after shampooing or as a curative measure between shampoos, with specially formulated products called *conditioners.* The purpose is to enhance and improve the appearance of the hair by adding luster, pliability, shine, softness and manageability.

Cortex: The second layer of the hair shaft, which contains the pigment that gives hair its color.

Cuticle: The outer, protective layer of the hair shaft, which is penetrated when permanent hair coloring is applied.

Demarcation: Also *regrowth* or *roots;* a visible line between lightened or tinted hair and the new growth of natural hair.

Developer: An agent—for example, hydrogen peroxide—that reacts chemically with coloring material to create a change in hair color.

Drab: To tone down or remove too-bright reds or brassy yellows while tinting or lightening.

Drabber: The agent used to diminish or remove too-warm tones (yellow, orange, brass).

Dye: An old-fashioned word to describe an outmoded product or preparation that permanently coats the hair shaft with artificial-looking color. Erroneously used as a synonym for *tint.*

Filler: A preparation designed to correct over-porosity in hair, thus allowing for more uniform coverage of the hair shafts in tinting and toning.

Frost: Also, *frosting.* To lighten numerous small strands of hair on the head to give a light, frosty look.

Gray: In nature, actually white hair (unpigmented) which gives the illusion of gray when scattered throughout the natural hair color.

Henna: This dye is extracted from a plant. Its use is revived from time to time, but it is little used now, since it coats the hair shaft with a permanent, often artificial-looking, bright shade of red. *White henna* is not henna, but magnesium carbonate, a harsh, highly alkaline bleaching agent that is little used because it ultimately damages the hair.

Highlighting: Subtle lightening and toning of hair to produce light-reflecting facets.

Lifting: Also, *lifting the color.* To lighten hair very slightly without effecting any color change.

Lightener: The chemical agent used to lighten the hair; it should (and usually does) contain conditioning substances.

Lightening: To remove pigment from the hair in order to make it lighter, paler. An old-fashioned word for this is "bleaching."

Long-lasting rinse: See *semipermanent coloring.*

Metallic salts: A residue, left by some temporary colors, which can affect the results of permanent waving or subsequent coloring.

Over-bleached: Refers to hair that has been excessively lightened or "bleached" with the wrong chemicals; also to hair exposed too often to too much sun and salt water. The condition is characterized by hair that is highly porous; it absorbs water too quickly and takes too long to dry. The hair looks dry and dull, with split or broken ends.

Overlap: Retinting (or relightening), during the process of retouching, of hair that has been previously colored or lightened.

Oxidation: Undesirable change in hair color due to the atmosphere or to water used in shampooing.

Painting: One of the most delicate ways to give highlights to hair, by brushing a mild lightener on selected strands.

Patch test: See *Allergy test.* So called because only a small area or "patch" of the skin is tested.

Penetrating color: The most widely used permanent hair coloring, so called because the color actually enters or penetrates the cortex or second layer of the hair shaft to change pigmentation.

Permanent color: Color that remains until the hair grows out and that cannot be shampooed out. See *Penetrating color.*

Peroxide: Actually hydrogen peroxide, one of the ingredients of hair lighteners.

Pigment: Color, natural or otherwise.

Porosity: In coloring or shampooing, the degree to which hair can absorb moisture—water or other liquids.

Powder bleach: An extremely fast-acting, strong bleach not now generally in use.

Prebleach: To prelighten the hair in preparation for toning and tinting with color. The purpose is to increase the porosity of the hair so that it will accept a tint or toning.

Prelighten: A more modern term for *prebleach.*

Presoften: An outmoded word for *prelighten.*

Remover: Also *Color remover.* A professional preparation for removing unwanted artificial color from the hair preparatory to applying fresh coloring, toning or lightening.

Resistant: Describes hair of low porosity which does not readily accept color.

Retouch: To lighten or color new growth on color-treated or lightened hair.

Rinse: Basically, two kinds—*semipermanent* and *temporary.* *Semipermanent rinse* is a preparation that imparts neither lasting color (see *Permanent color*) nor color which can be removed by shampooing; the color fades gradually over a period of several weeks. Also referred to as a *toner* or color *lotion. Temporary rinse* is applied after shampooing, to add color, which is deposited on the surface of the hair shaft and can be removed immediately by shampooing the hair.

Roots: In reference to tinted or lightened hair, this is simply new growth, which shows the natural color of the hair.

Semipermanent color: See *Rinse.*

Shade: A color; also a gradation of color, as in "will lighten two or three shades."

Shampoo tint: A shampoo or cleansing agent mixed with coloring substances, which is applied like a shampoo.

Shampoo for colored or tinted hair: See *Colorfast shampoo.*

Skin test: See *Allergy test;* also, *Patch test.*

Strand test: See *Color test.*

Strand: A small section of hair, forty to sixty hairs.

Streak: An area of the hair that is noticeably lighter than the rest of the hair; also, to lighten small groups of strands, usually at the hairline.

Strip: To use a remover to take out artificial color in the hair; a corrective procedure in most cases.

Temporary color: A color that may be removed immediately from the hair by shampooing.

Tint: A permanent hair coloring that cannot be shampooed out and remains until the hair grows out, unless it is chemically removed. The agent penetrates the hair shaft and alters the pigmentation of the cortex.

Tip: To lighten the ends of strands of hair, to contrast strongly or subtly with the other, darker hair.

Tone: A color that modifies another one—e.g., brunette hair with an overall red "tone"; also, a way of designating color value—e.g., a warm "tone" of blonde.

Touch up: See *Retouch.*

Vegetable color: A temporary color made from the pigments of various plants; a color that coats and does not penetrate the hair shaft.

Virgin hair: Hair that has never been altered by lightening, tinting, permanenting or relaxing.

Warm: A descriptive word for any hair color that contains red or gold tones.

Index

ABOUT THE AUTHOR

Leslie Blanchard, whose name is synonymous throughout the world with beautiful hair color, is one of the most vital personalities in the business.

The Private World of Leslie Blanchard, the quietly luxurious salon he established in 1970 in his townhouse on New York's East Sixty-second Street, is a mecca for socialites, celebrities and others wise to where the art of hair coloring and hair care has reached its apogee. Regular enthusiasts include Barbara Walters, Ellen Burstyn, Cheryl Tiegs, Meryl Streep, Nancy Allen, Mary Tyler Moore and a host of top New York models. Robert De Niro and Donald Sutherland are among the male Hollywood luminaries on Leslie's long list of devotees. In addition, there doesn't seem to be a blonde in America who doesn't admire his talent.

Leslie arrived in New York from his native Barre, Vermont, after training in Boston. He joined Elizabeth Arden and later became color director of Saks Fifth Avenue's New York salon. During this period, he was appointed senior color consultant for Clairol, a post he still holds.

Since the start of his career, color has been Leslie's absorbing interest. He is famous for taking the brassiness out of blondeness, and for giving hair coloring "believability," with a natural mingling of shades that improve on nature the way skillfully applied makeup does.

Leslie believes that hair coloring must relate to current fashion, and seldom misses the New York and Paris fashion openings. His reputation as an astute and level-headed businessman, along with the magic of his name and talents, are now channeled into wider fields. He has created his own collection of specially formulated hair-care products, which are available at stores throughout the country.

Included are all the essentials—shampoos, conditioners, revitalizing lotion, moisturizing hair cream, setting lotion and finishing spray.

Leslie's spare time is divided between his Manhattan and Beverly Hills apartments, filled, like his salon, with a profusion of fresh-cut flowers, and his hundred-acre Yellow Iris Farm in New Jersey, where he breeds prize-winning Morgan horses. He's also a passionate gardener, a compulsive traveler, a collector of Mexican paintings and of American folk art, and a tireless host who, with the help of his Chinese cook, offers some of the most sought-after dinner invitations in town.

Leslie is a charmer, a realist, a sage and, as his many interviewers have discovered, a headline maker. In addition, the quality and amiability of his personality have earned him devotion from both his clientele and the people with whom he is closely associated. He loves life, and his work—and it shows.